WOMAN TO WOMAN

WOMAN TO WOMAN

A Leading Gynecologist Tells You
All You Need to Know About Your
Body And Your Health

❧

Yvonne S. Thornton, M.D., M.P.H.
with Jo Coudert

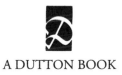

A DUTTON BOOK

This book is dedicated to my professors

Thomas F. Dillon, M.D.

who gave me the opportunity to realize my dream
of becoming an obstetrician

and

Edward T. Bowe, M.D.

whose practice of obstetrics and gynecology
should stand as a beacon to all
who enter the field of health care for women

DUTTON
Published by the Penguin Group
Penguin Books USA Inc., 375 Hudson Street,
New York, New York 10014, U.S.A.
Penguin Books Ltd, 27 Wrights Lane,
London W8 5TZ, England
Penguin Books Australia Ltd, Ringwood,
Victoria, Australia
Penguin Books Canada Ltd, 10 Alcorn Avenue,
Toronto, Ontario, Canada M4V 3B2
Penguin Books (N.Z.) Ltd, 182–190 Wairau Road,
Auckland 10, New Zealand

Penguin Books Ltd, Registered Offices:
Harmondsworth, Middlesex, England

First published by Dutton, an imprint of Dutton Signet,
a division of Penguin Books USA Inc.
Distributed in Canada by McClelland & Stewart Inc.

First Printing, August, 1997
10 9 8 7 6 5 4 3 2 1

LIBRARY OF CONGRESS CATALOGING-IN-PUBLICATION DATA: is available

ISBN: 0-525-94297-1

Printed in the United States of America
Set in Janson Text
Designed by Leonard Telesca

A NOTE TO THE READER
The ideas, procedures, and suggestions contained in this book are not intended as a substitute for medical treatment by a physician. The reader should regularly consult a physician in matters relating to health.

PUBLISHER'S NOTE

CONTENTS

FOREWORD

The amount of information that health care professionals need to carry in their proverbial "doctor's bag" is burgeoning. Concurrently, women patients are more aware of their health needs and are demanding more information about their body systems and functions. Unfortunately, many gaps, misinformation, and myths are widespread, especially regarding the female reproductive system.

Dr. Yvonne Thornton has taken on the task of dispelling these myths. And she is superbly qualified to inform and clarify. A "first" in many instances, she was the first in her family to go to medical school; the first black woman to go into academic gynecology; and the first black woman gynecologist to become director of a division in the Department of Obstetrics and Gynecology on the faculty of The New York Hospital-Cornell Medical Center.

Her excellent teaching capabilities stand her in good stead as she continues to teach, in the present case her patients and women at large. She demystifies the female reproductive system and its functions with grace and a sense of humor. And a lesson learned with laughter is a lesson well remembered.

Lila Wallis, M.D., M.A.C.P.
Clinical Professor of Medicine,
    Cornell University Medical College
Attending Physician, The New York Hospital

Former President,
    American Medical Women's Association
Founding President,
    National Council on Women's Health

PREFACE

Growing up as one of six girls in my family, I had a natural curiosity about the female reproductive tract. I listened to my mother, sisters, aunts, and classmates, storing up all the mysteries and myths I overheard, only to discover upon entering medical school that many of the most widely held beliefs about women's health care were, at best, inaccurate and, at worst, potentially harmful, even life-threatening. Explaining what the facts actually were to my sisters and working-class parents helped me develop straightforward communicative skills that later proved invaluable in my professional role as a physician and obstetrician-gynecologist.

Because I am a woman and a mother as well as a physician, I have been on both sides of the stirrups. During my ten years of general OB/GYN faculty practice at The New York Hospital-Cornell Medical Center, I came to understand women's concerns, their wish for solid, accurate information and their need for comfort and reassurance. Both then and now as a specialist in perinatalogy, I find myself saying, "Let me tell you what this really means" or "Let me tell you what really happens" or "Let me explain why this procedure is necessary." I am not impatient when a woman expresses her belief that the placenta is attached to the navel or that because she has had a hysterectomy, she does not need a pelvic exam. Even in this enlightened age, I still encounter misconceptions daily, even among the most educated women, which is why I decided there was a need for a comprehensive, readable book covering *both* obstetrics and gynecology.

Because of menstruation, pregnancy, childbirth, and menopause, a woman is necessarily more involved with her body than a man is with his. I believe it is important that she understand how it works, how best to care for it, and how to make sensible decisions concerning it. Because she is the person living in her body, she is the one who can detect any change promptly, which makes her the first line of defense where her gynecologic and reproductive health is concerned. Good and useful information allows a woman to know when to seek treatment and to act as a partner with her gynecologist in the detection and handling of problems. It also enables her to deal optimally with the different stages of life as they come along.

This book is intended to address the concerns voiced by a cross-section of women while, at the same time, dispelling the myths and misconceptions that have plagued women throughout the centuries. Hopefully, after reading this book, girls and women—and men, too, if they are interested—will have greatly added to their knowledge about the female body, enabling them to make informed choices and decisions about their health care.

Knowledge is always useful; knowledge about the female self can be life-enhancing—and sometimes life-saving. This is why I am pleased to share with you the following journey through the world of femaleness.

Yvonne S. Thornton, M.D., M.P.H.

I

THE WORKS

1

THE FEMININE PHYSIQUE

❧

THE WORKS • OVARIES • FALLOPIAN TUBES • UTERUS • CERVIX • VAGINA AND VULVA • BREASTS • THE BOSSES • PITUITARY • HYPOTHALAMUS • THE WORKING OF THE WORKS • MENSTRUATION • WHAT IS A NORMAL PERIOD? • KEEPING A MENSTRUAL CHART • MITTELSCHMERZ • WHEN A PERIOD BECOMES A QUESTION MARK • AMEN-ORRHEA • OLIGOMENORRHEA • POLYMENORRHEA • DYSMENORRHEA • CLOTS • REGULATION OF PERIODS • BIRTH CONTROL PILLS • DIAGNOSTIC PROCEDURES • PMS—FACTS AND FICTIONS • TO DOUCHE OR NOT TO DOUCHE • DOUCHING TO PREVENT PREGNANCY • PAINFUL INTERCOURSE • LUBRICATION • INFECTION • AGE •

The basic anatomy of the human female is a mystery to many women. Even highly educated and sophisticated women may not know the difference between a urethra and a ureter. A patient of mine, a lawyer, was surprised to learn that her fallopian tubes were not attached to her navel when we discussed the procedure of tubal ligation, that is, the tying of her tubes, after she delivered her third child. Let us attempt to clear up any possible confusion by taking a tour of the female reproductive organs.

THE WORKS

Ovaries. The ovaries are two firm, walnut-sized structures sus-pended from either side of the uterus. Dull white and bumpy in appearance, they produce the hormones estrogen and progesterone. Eggs are stored inside the ovaries, and every month, in a process called ovulation, one of the ovaries releases an egg, or ovum, the size of a sugar granule. First, an egg sac called a follicle develops inside the ovary in response to follicle-stimulating hormone (FSH), and when the follicle ruptures on command of certain other hormones, the egg is released.

A female is born with all the eggs she will ever have; no more will be produced in her lifetime. When a female fetus is twenty weeks old, the ovaries contain six million eggs. This is their peak number. By the time the baby girl is born, the number of eggs is already down to two million. By adolescence, 300,000 eggs remain, and when that girl becomes a 36-year-old woman, only 34,000 eggs remain. Luckily, women require no more than about 400 eggs throughout their entire reproductive lives, suggesting that the much, much larger number of eggs available is a fail-safe mechanism on the part of Mother Nature.

Fallopian Tubes. There are two fallopian tubes. Each extends from the top of the uterus to form a passageway for the egg to travel from the ovary to the uterus. Although usually pictured as standing out in a T formation from the uterus, the fallopian tubes actually droop behind

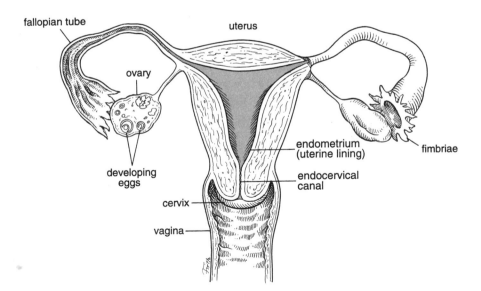

The Female Reproductive System

the uterus, hanging in a limp fashion with fingerlike projections (fimbriae) at the ends. These fimbriae sweep over the surface of the ovaries at regular intervals, and when an egg is released from an ovary, the fimbriae on that side vacuum up the egg. The egg then travels down the fallopian tube into the uterus, where, if it has been fertilized, it is implanted.

If a patient of mine has difficulty envisioning the spatial relationship of the fallopian tubes to the uterus, I am apt to impersonate the two by standing with my arms hanging loosely behind me. My body then represents the uterus, my arms the fallopian tubes, and my fingers the fimbriae.

Uterus. Often referred to as the womb, the uterus is the "storage facility" for the fetus in a normal pregnancy. It is divided into two unequal parts, with the larger part being the body, or fundus, while the smaller is the cervix, or neck. The lining of the uterus, which is called the endometrium, undergoes change in accordance with changing levels of circulating hormones. Right after a menstrual period, the endometrium can be as thin as indoor-outdoor carpeting, while at midcycle it is as plushly luxuriant as a velvety Oriental rug. When this endometrial lining is sloughed off each month, the resulting blood flow is referred to as menstruation. As well as blood, the menstrual flow contains tiny fragments of shed uterine lining.

Cervix. The cervix is that part of the uterus (the neck) that is connected to the vagina. It feels like a bump at the top of the vagina and is as firm as a nose. The cervix produces mucus, and this mucus changes consistency in response to hormones, particularly estrogen. Just prior to ovulation the mucus is thin and elastic so as to allow sperm from the male easier access to the womb. At other times it is thick and less penetrable.

An internal os, or mouth, at one end of the cervix opens into the body of the uterus, and an external os at the opposite end opens into the vagina. These openings act like doors. After childbearing, the external os may remain ajar, but the internal os is characteristically closed. The corridor between the two is known as the endocervical canal, and it and the external os are important in gynecology because it is here that cell samples are collected for a Pap smear. The internal os, on the other hand, is important in obstetrics because a mucus plug in this area prevents bacteria from ascending into the womb and infecting the fetus.

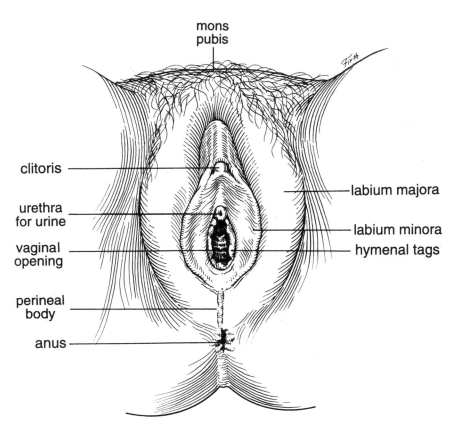

mons pubis

clitoris

urethra for urine

vaginal opening

perineal body

anus

labium majora

labium minora

hymenal tags

External Female Genitalia

Vagina and Vulva. The vagina is a tubular structure linking the uterus to the outside world of the vulva. It accommodates the male organ during intercourse, and during childbirth it is the birth canal through which the baby enters the world. In the young female, before intercourse has occurred, the entrance of the vagina is partially covered by a membrane called the hymen. Initial intercourse tears the hymen, leaving tags of tissue behind. Because the tearing is rather like a fist going through a bass drum, the process can be painful and bleeding usually occurs.

The vulva includes all structures visible on the outside, from the fat-filled cushion covering the pubic bone, known as the mons pubis, to the anus. The external female genitalia include the clitoris, the labia majora and labia minora, and the urethra. The labia, so called from the Latin word for "lips," are the inner and outer folds of skin enclosing the clitoris, urethra, vagina, and the perineal body, which is the area between the vagina and the anus.

When a woman is lying on her back, uppermost is the clitoris, which is analogous to the penis in the male and is the prime organ of sexual sensation. Next comes the urethra through which urine flows from the bladder to the outside. Just below the urethra is the vagina, and the last opening farther down is the anus. Figure 2 shows why it is important, after urinating, to wipe from the front to the back rather than the reverse; the anus is filled with bacteria that can cause a bladder infection if allowed to gain entry through the urethra.

Breasts. The breasts are mammary (milk-producing) glands responsive to hormones released during the monthly cycle and after childbirth. When the breasts are producing milk, this process is called lactation.

THE BOSSES

The breasts, ovaries, and uterus are referred to as end-organs, that is, their workings are dictated by chemical messengers coming from other organs, in this case the pituitary gland and the hypothalamus, both of which are situated in the head.

Pituitary. The pituitary gland is an endocrine organ, that is, an organ that secrets substances into the blood which have a specific effect on other organs. The larger part of the pituitary, the anterior lobe, comes from the same tissue as the pharynx, which is the tube connecting the mouth and the esophagus. The smaller part, the posterior lobe, is formed from the floor of the hypothalamus in the brain. It sits immediately beneath the brain and is connected to it by a stalk.

The pituitary secretes follicle-stimulating hormone (FSH) in response to low or declining levels of circulating estrogen and progesterone. The FSH stimulates egg follicles to grow and compete to become the large follicle holding the egg that will be released from the ovary at midcycle (ovulation). As midcycle approaches, the level of estrogen increases, which in turn shuts off FSH and prompts a rise in another pituitary hormone, luteinizing hormone (LH). This hormone stimulates release of the egg from the ovary, usually at midcycle. The ruptured follicle left behind is called the corpus luteum

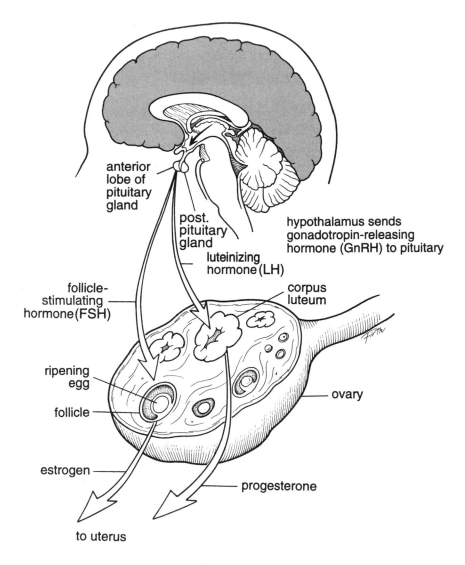

anterior
lobe of
pituitary
gland

post.
pituitary
gland

luteinizing
hormone (LH)

hypothalamus sends
gonadotropin-releasing
hormone (GnRH) to pituitary

follicle-
stimulating
hormone (FSH)

corpus
luteum

ripening
egg

follicle

ovary

estrogen

progesterone

to uterus

The Bosses

(yellow body). This corpus luteum secretes a hormone called progesterone. Progesterone, in concert with estrogen, prepares the
uterine lining to nourish the fertilized egg. If the egg is not fertilized, the corpus luteum degenerates over the next 14 days, a process
that both signals the uterine lining to slough off (menstruation) and
triggers a rise in the level of FSH, and the whole cycle starts over
again.

Hypothalamus. This organ, situated in the brain, is the ultimate boss. It produces gonadotropin-releasing hormone (GnRH), which stimulates the pituitary to release FSH and LH, and these in turn stimulate the production of estrogen and progesterone by the ovaries.

THE WORKING OF THE WORKS

In young girls the first signs of maturation occur in the nipples and breast tissue. This stage is called the thelarche, from the Greek word for nipple. Sometimes as early as six years of age but usually around ten, girls start developing little mounds on their chest, and mothers who observe these "mosquito bites" note to themselves that the menarche, the establishment of menstruation, cannot be too far off. An intermediate stage comes before the menarche, however. Known as the pubarche, this stage occurs about a year after breast tissue begins to develop and is characterized by the appearance of hair in the pubic area and under the arms. It is another year or so after this that menstruation commences.

Menstruation. The average age of the onset of menstruation is 12.6 to 12.8 years, with the range being from 9.1 to 17.7 years. Mothers tell me about daughters going on 11 who expect to have their periods by the time they are 12. The day after their twelfth birthday they are saying, "Mommy, Mommy, Joanie has her period. How come I don't have mine?" What they don't realize is that 12 years and 8 months is almost 13 years and they are jumping the gun a bit. But I must admit this is preferable to earlier times when mothers were too reticent to prepare their daughters for what was coming. All too many girls, out climbing trees with their brothers, suddenly feared they were bleeding to death and entered womanhood on a shock wave of dismay.

Some girls who are thin do not have their periods until they have reached a critical body weight, others not until they are 16 or even 18 years old. Although these ages are still within the normal range, albeit at the upper limit, either peer pressure or a nervous mother is likely to have landed the girl in a gynecologist's office by the time she is 14 or 15. The advice she receives then will probably be to wait and see. Only when absolutely nothing has happened by age 16 does the possibility of a hormonal problem need to be investigated.

What Is a Normal Period? Periods (menses) are irregular in 50 percent of adolescent girls. A period may come once and then not again for another six months, or come once every three months, or skip back and forth between once a month and once every two or three months. Bleeding may be light one month and heavy the next, and it may last for two days or five days. All sorts of variations from what adult women experience as normal are common because it can take time for the hormones to become regulated. But eventually they do settle down and a pattern is established.

The normal cycle is said to be 28 days, the length of the lunar (not the calendar) month, but variations on "normal" are legion. Seldom in my experience as a gynecologist have I encountered a person with a 28-day cycle. I am much more used to hearing 30 days, 26 days, 40 days, even once every two months or, rarely, three months.

"Normal," then, is what is normal for the particular individual. After the hormones have settled down and the periods are coming regularly, whether the pattern is every 28 days, every 40 days, or every two months, when it has persisted for a couple of years, it is clear that is that particular female's cycle; it is normal for her.

If the cycle is longer than 28 days, the variation in time comes prior to ovulation because after ovulation occurs, it is always, in every woman, 13 to 15 days until the start of the next period. With a 28-day cycle, 14 days will be preovulatory; with a 40-day cycle, 26 of those days will be preovulatory. This is important to know if pregnancy is desired, as I found out when I wanted to get pregnant; I had a 40-day cycle, so I was ovulating on day 26, not on day 14 as the textbooks have it.

Keeping a Menstrual Chart. Not only is there variation in cyclicity among women, but the timing of cycles does not necessarily remain the same throughout the 35 to 40 years a woman menstruates. A woman in her 20's may menstruate every 32 days, then she enters her 30's and her periods come every 26 days, and after 35 she may go to 40 days. Although the change should be investigated, if a new regularity becomes established, then it is clear that a new phase has been entered.

A woman herself is her own best control, that is, she should compare herself with herself. What matters after a pattern has been established is whether there is any change in it. To this end, every female,

Menstrual Cycle

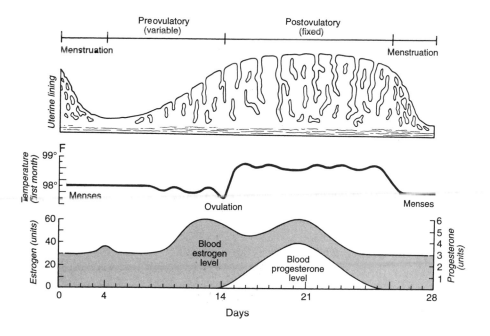

Interrelationship of Hormones, Body Temperature,
Ovulation and Menstruation

when she starts menstruating, should keep a chart. The type illustrated works well because marking the squares to indicate a period allows any deviation in timing to become immediately apparent.

When a woman comes to me with a report of menstrual irregularities, I say, "Let's look at your menstrual calendar. Okay, it was every 26 days up till here, and then what happened?"

She may answer, "That's about the time I started horseback riding." Or "I wanted to lose weight and went on a near-starvation diet." Or "I fell in love and began having intercourse." Any one of these can be a sufficient explanation—but only after other possible causes have been ruled out in a process known as diagnosis by exclusion.

If I see from her calendar that 40 days have gone by, pregnancy is the first possibility to be excluded. I ask the woman if she is sexually active, and I explain that "sexually active" means any

Menstrual Calendar

	1	2	3	4	5	6	7	8	9	10	11	12	13	14	15	16	17	18	19	20	21	22	23	24	25	26	27	28	29	30	31
Jan.	B	B	B	B	S	S				I																					
Feb.	B	B	B	B	S	S			I																						
Mar.							B	B	B	B	S	S																			
Apr.	S	S														I															
May																															
June																															
July																															
Aug.																															
Sep.																															
Oct.																															
Nov.																															
Dec.																															

S=spotting   B=bleeding   I=intercourse

exposure to sperm. It does not have to be complete intercourse. It can be "just outside, he didn't come in." If by this or any other definition the woman is sexually active, then a pregnancy test is in order.

If the pregnancy test is negative or if the woman is not sexually active, I proceed to rule out other possible causes, such as a sudden sizable weight gain or loss or a marked increased in physical activity, such as going into training as a runner. When no such explanation exists, I suggest to the woman that our best course is to wait for another cycle to see whether a change in periodicity is establishing itself.

"You're 30 now," I say. "When you're 35, it may change again." Although this change in periodicity is not described in textbooks, I have seen it over and over in my practice, so frequently that it cannot be abnormal. As far as I am aware, no studies have been done, no statistics gathered, perhaps because nobody thinks it worth bothering about, but I know from my own experience that a lengthening or shortening of the cycle often occurs, and I have the impression that the ages ending in zero or five—20, 25, 30, 35, 40—seem to be involved most often.

Having this bit of information does not mean, however, that a woman should shrug off a deviation in her cycle. While it is likely to have a benign explanation, any change in cyclicity should send a woman to her gynecologist promptly. This is why keeping a menstrual chart is important: It acts as an early warning system for the woman, alerting her to seek medical attention, and it is a visual aid for the doctor that is far more informative than a vague statement such as, "My periods seem to be getting more frequent."

Mittelschmerz. Another advantage of keeping a menstrual chart is that it identifies the time of ovulation, which occurs at the midpoint of the cycle. When the egg ruptures through the ovary, there can be an imbalance in estrogen and progesterone levels, and that may in turn affect the lining of the uterus, causing it to slough off a little bit of blood. This slight discharge is known as *mittelschmerz*, German for "a pain in the middle," although it is more graphic to think of it as a "schmear in the middle."

When an anxious patient says, "I'm bleeding every other day now," and I ask her when it started and she answers, "October fourteenth," if I look at her menstrual calendar and find that October 14 is right at midcycle, I am relieved. I know it is mittelschmerz and nothing to be concerned about.

The same is true if the discharge is white or pale yellow. The vagina as well as the uterus may respond to the midcycle surge in hormones with an increased discharge. Patients come to my office complaining, "Oh, the discharge is so heavy. Something must be terribly wrong." I ask for the date of the first day of their last period, and if the discharge is particularly noticeable at midcycle, I reassure them that it is not something to be concerned about. "I'll take a culture," I say, "to make sure it's not chlamydia and not infectious, but nine chances out of ten it's only mittelschmerz."

WHEN A PERIOD BECOMES A QUESTION MARK

Amenorrhea. There is primary amenorrhea, which is no periods at all by age 16, and secondary amenorrhea, which is cessation of already established menses, the latter being by far the most common. If the periods have ceased and the patient is not pregnant, a hormonal imbalance is the most likely explanation. If the patient is an adolescent, I inquire into whether she has been losing weight or is distressed. Usually it turns out that she has been on a diet and lost 35 pounds, or she has gone away to boarding school for the first time, or her parents are in the midst of a divorce and there is a great deal of stress in her life.

Stress can cause the periods to cease in adults as well as adolescents. But amenorrhea should not be assumed to be due to stress without a physical examination to eliminate other causes. Nor should the amenorrhea be allowed to go beyond three months because when the woman finally does have her period, it is likely to be a dangerously heavy bleed. Estrogen has been affecting the lining of the uterus, making the endometrium nice and plump, and those growing cells need to be sloughed off. When they are not, when the uterus has been stimulated for so long without shedding, the woman may end up in the hospital with a hemorrhage.

Oligomenorrhea. While amenorrhea is the absence of menses, oligomenorrhea is defined as abnormally infrequent or scanty menstruation, and the same considerations apply. It must be medically evaluated to try to pin down the cause, and steps must be taken to correct it to obviate the risk of the growing cells piling up in the uterine lining.

Oligomenorrhea followed by amenorrhea for several months in a woman in her late 40's is usually the first sign that she is entering menopause.

Polymenorrhea. At the opposite extreme is the situation where periods are coming every two to three weeks. This type of irregular bleeding, be it in an adolescent, a 25-year-old, or a 55-year-old, must be evaluated promptly to rule out polyps or any other abnormal condition that may be causing the polymenorrhea. When the uterine tissue has been biopsied and found to be normal, then we assume the dysfunction has to do with hormonal regulation. But we cannot then go on to say that the cause is an overactive or underactive pituitary gland or some other imbalance because the truth is that we do not know. The old term for polymenorrhea was *dysfunctional uterine bleeding*, but that was just a more high-sounding way of saying the cause is unknown.

Dysmenorrhea. Dysmenorrhea, or cramps, is colicky pain or discomfort in the mid or lower abdomen, perhaps radiating to the lower back and legs, experienced with a period. The cause of cramps is thought to be contractions of the uterus as the lining is being sloughed off, with the contractions being a direct effect of prostaglandin on the uterine muscle. (Prostaglandin, present in the uterine lining, is a substance that causes muscle contractions.) Although most women have cramping during their menses, the abdominal symptoms are usually mild and subside within a few days after the beginning of the menstrual flow. If this is not the case and the cramps progress to severe or unrelenting pain, the term dysmenorrhea is applied and the condition calls for medical evaluation and treatment. The nonsteroidal anti-inflammatory drugs such as aspirin, ibuprofen, naprosyn, and mefe-namicacid (Ponstel) block the prostaglandins from exerting their cramping effect and provide relief of mild to severe menstrual cramps.

Clots. A patient will arrive at my office thoroughly upset because "My period's coming out in clots." I ask how big the clots are, and if she tells me they are anything smaller than a piece of liver and are not soaking an external pad in an hour, I tell her not to worry about them. I explain that endometrial lining of the uterus gets plush and succulent and thick under the influence of estrogen. If progesterone is not secreted in timely fashion to counteract the estrogen, the lining continues to thicken and may start breaking off in pieces. The longer the time between periods, the more likely this is to occur, which is why progesterone is often prescribed for patients whose periods are delayed or widely spaced to stabilize the endometrium and ensure that the bleed will be orderly.

Even in a normal period there will be blood clots because it is vascular tissue that is being shed, but the actual pieces of endometrium tend to be microscopic and most women do not notice them. Since they are particularly likely to emerge when the toilet is being used, they are simply flushed away. New pads will sometimes show bits of clot; if the pads have webbing on the outside, some tissue may remain on top while the blood soaks through to the layers beneath. The only time to be concerned about clots is when excessive bleeding soaks an external pad with bright red blood and the pad needs to be changed every hour.

REGULATION OF PERIODS

Birth Control Pills. Many gynecologists prescribe birth control pills for women with polymenorrhea on the theory that the steady supply of estrogen and progesterone the pills provide will make up for any hormonal imbalance. A course of low-dose birth control pills stabilizes the endometrial lining and allows it to build up. The pills are used for three to six months; after they are discontinued, the periods usually respond by coming regularly again.

It is a different story, however, if, in an attempt to regulate her cycle, birth control pills are prescribed for the woman whose periods come only every two or three months. Obviously, the hypothalamus and pituitary with their control mechanisms for the period are not functioning at 100 percent. They may be functioning at 85 percent, which is not a problem; it only means that the period comes every eight weeks instead of every four. However, many doctors feel that a woman must have a period every 28 days and prescribe birth control pills to make certain she does.

The woman dutifully follows a regimen of 21 hormone pills a month and the pills take over the prerogatives of the hypothalamus and pituitary, in effect putting them to sleep. Now it is the birth control pills that are dictating the cycle, causing an artificial period, and when the woman stops taking them after six months or so, she may never have a period again.

I have had any number of women come to my office saying, "I was having periods every two months and my gynecologist wanted to regulate me so he put me on the Pill. I took it for a year and then I stopped because I want to have a baby, and now my periods don't come at all." I explain that the little pituitary and hypothalamus glands that were struggling along every two months got sat on by the Pill and now cannot get themselves cranked up again. (For the treatment of anovulatory cycles, see chapter 7.)

Diagnostic Procedures. Heavy or irregular bleeding (menorrhagia), periods that are coming without rhyme or reason, warrant careful investigation by means of an endometrial biopsy. This can be done in the gynecologist's office. A scoop-shaped plastic catheter called a curette is inserted into the uterus to scrape off a sample of the endometrial lining. With training and experience the gynecologist becomes skilled at judging the feel of the endometrial cavity, whether it is irregular or jagged, whether there are things like polyps growing in there or whether the lining is clumped to one side. Sometimes a polyp comes out in the sampling pass made with the curette, or a polyp may be hanging outside the cervix like a tongue and the gynecologist can just grasp it and remove it.

The tissue removed is sent to a pathology laboratory for examina-

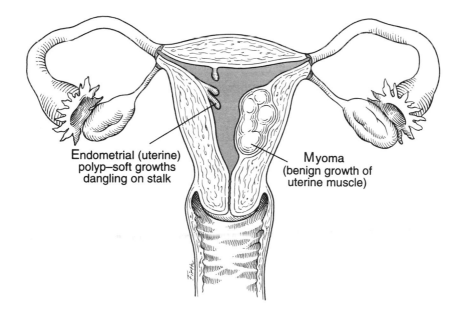

Myoma and Polyps in Uterus

tion. A concern with endometrial sampling is that the gynecologist may be taking a sample on the right side of the uterus, for instance, and missing cancerous changes on the left; but if malignancy is present, it is usually throughout the uterus, and in general, office biopsies are very good at providing a diagnosis. Sometimes they even prove remedial: The pass with the curette smooths the endometrial lining or removes the polyp, and the irregular bleeding ceases. However, if the procedure yields no results, a formal D and C—dilatation and curettage of the uterus—is the next step. The patient often protests, "Why didn't you do that in the first place?" My answer is that I want to see if I can obtain a diagnosis without having to resort to a more involved procedure. Even though a D and C is probably the most frequently performed of all operative procedures and is viewed as routine, I consider that whenever a patient goes to the operating room, there is always the potential, however slight, of a mishap. In a D and C there can be perforation of the uterus or complications from the anesthesia, and I prefer to avoid the risk if I can get the same information from an office procedure.

If heavy bleeding continues despite the office procedure, one polyp may have been removed but another missed, or the lining of the uterus is clumped to one side, or a submucous myoma has indented the lining. Most myomas grow on the outside of the uterus like Mickey Mouse ears, but some grow inside, making the endometrial lining irregular and causing a disruption in the menstrual sloughing-off process (see chapter 16).

A D and C is done in the hospital in a same-day procedure—in by nine, out by five, like dry cleaning. It is done under heavy sedation or light general anesthesia. When the patient regains consciousness, she is likely to be experiencing cramps because there has been instrumentation in the uterus, but medication will ameliorate them. She will need someone, however, to escort her home.

A D and C is designed to be both diagnostic and therapeutic. The cervix is first dilated (stretched) in order to accommodate the curette, and curettage smooths the lining, making it clean and even. If the physician finds it necessary to inspect the inside of the uterus visually, a hysteroscope—a long, thin instrument much like a telescope—is used. When the presence of a myoma is noted within the uterine cavity, a more sophisticated and involved procedure than a D and C is carried out at a later date, or if the tissue obtained is diagnosed as malignant on laboratory examination, the patient will be referred to a cancer specialist.

PMS—FACTS AND FICTIONS

At midcycle there is a sudden surge in hormonal release because the body is getting ready for pregnancy. If the egg is fertilized, large amounts of hormones are needed to support the base mechanism of the growing placenta, but if the egg is not fertilized, the woman is stuck with the excess hormones and PMS, or premenstrual syndrome, is the result. Women respond to it in different ways: Some get bloated, some experience supercharged emotions, some erupt in acne because they have receptors for the hormones in their faces. There is even a rare condition called catamenial pneumothorax in which receptors in the lungs respond to the surge of hormones and blood vessels rupture, causing breathing difficulties. The woman who knows that her body responds to the hormone surge in this way

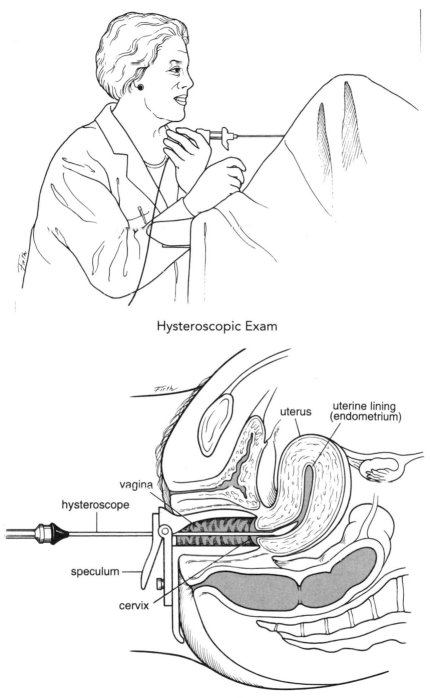

Hysteroscopic Exam

hysteroscope

vagina

uterus

uterine lining
(endometrium)

speculum

cervix

Hysteroscope within Uterus

learns to take it in stride. After the initial "Eek!" she says, "Oh, it's just my lung again. It's midcycle."

Some women have no perceptible reaction. Of those who do, the majority handle it the same way they handle their period; they know it is coming and adjust their activities accordingly. But some women—not a large number—become emotionally disturbed. This does not mean that their hormone release is greater but that they react more sensitively to it. If a woman is by nature somewhat depressive or somewhat manic, what is already there as a matrix becomes amplified. This leads some people to believe that all women are crazy or have mood swings, but this is not so, nor is it justified to say, "Oh, my God, she's suffering from PMS. Better watch out." It just means that women who are borderline manic-depressive may have their condition exacerbated.

The problem in treating PMS is that the symptoms are not necesssarily all the same. Ms. X can have one set of symptoms, Ms. Y another, and the treatment that works with one will not work with the other. The physician who grows frustrated with the failure of his or her approach may resort to saying, "It's all in your head." But women need not—indeed, should not—accept this dictum. PMS is real. It exists. It is more prominent in some patients than others, but every woman has the potential of having severe PMS because of the physiologic surge in hormones.

I suspect that how a woman copes with it, whether she tells herself that she knows it is coming and just rides it out or whether she uses it as an excuse, depends somewhat on her mindset. But I could be wrong. There are still a lot of unknowns about PMS. We as physicians are placed in the position of being expected to know everything, and people do not like to accept that we do not—nor, for that matter, do some physicians. Patients look to us for answers, but sometimes we have to give advice based on nothing but our own experience, not on studies or investigations or experiments—which is certainly true in the case of PMS, where there is no single classic treatment approach to a classic set of symptoms.

The customary advice is: Get the sleep you need—at least seven and a half hours a night. Stay away from stressful situations. Don't eat refined sugar or chocolate. Exercise regularly. Know your own body, and try to formulate ways of dealing with PMS because if you don't, you are going to be debilitated for one week out of every month for 35 years. This counsel is not much consolation for the woman whose breasts and nipples become so sensitive that she cannot wear a sweater and would prefer not to have to answer the phone. But it is the best we can offer.

One patient to whom I said something of this nature startled me by bursting out, "Gee, I hate female impersonators! If a man is going to impersonate a woman, he should have PMS, cramps, bleeding— he should have everything I go through before he has a right to dress up, put on makeup, and look pretty. It's not fair!" She had a point. But, then, whoever said life was fair?

TO DOUCHE OR NOT TO DOUCHE

An axiom handed down from mother to daughter through the ages is that females have to douche; to keep clean, they must douche after menstruation and after intercourse. When I ask women their views on this, ninety-nine out of a hundred answer, "Oh, I have to douche. Definitely. I gotta." When I ask why, they say, "Because I've always done it, my mother's always done it, my grandmother's always done it." Douching is entrenched in female mores, perhaps in response to the ancient Biblical stigma of women being unclean, and despite any number of conclusive studies, women still carry on with this archaic, antiquated, and potentially dangerous procedure.

Nobody tells them that douching is unnecessary and harmful, certainly not the manufacturer who prospers financially by selling douche products. The only hope is for women to rise up and say, "What are we doing to ourselves? Let's question this." Douching should be like tonsillectomies. There was a time when every child had a tonsillectomy, until finally people said, "Wait a minute. Why are we doing this?" Sure enough, when studies were done, it turned out that every kid did not need a tonsillectomy. It is time we learned the same thing about douching.

When a patient says she douches "to make myself feel better, cleaner," I ask, "Is there an odor or something that makes you feel you have to douche?"

"No, it's just that when my period is over, I want to rinse out whatever is left there."

"That's logical, but do you know that your body does that? That's why you change your panties every day and throw them away after a while—because of a discharge, a natural discharge."

Bodies function excellently to take care of themselves. When menstruation ends, the 23 kinds of bacteria that are normally present in the vagina do the cleaning up. Just like the bacteria in the mouth and in the rectum, they are there for a reason: to keep the area tidy and ride herd on invaders. Furthermore, in the average woman the pH of the vagina is four. The pH of the stomach is one because of the hydrochloric acid in it, the pH of water is seven, so the pH of the vagina is in the middle, slightly on the acidic side, where it needs to remain in order to provide the right environment for the cleansing bacteria. With douching, that natural balance is disrupted. The vagina has to try to repair itself and get back to that pH of four, and the bacteria that have been washed out by the douching have to try to grow and reestablish themselves; sometimes, before that can happen, fungus starts to move in.

Fungus, or yeast, is not bacteria. In fact, it is the bacteria that keep fungus under control. Erase the bacteria by douching and all of a sudden the fungus is saying, "Hey, fellas, come on in. There's nobody here." And more and more fungus moves into the vagina and happily multiplies. What does fungus do? It causes a tremendous itch and a tremendous discharge, and the woman is quickly going out of her mind. Thinking it will help, she douches again, and the three or four little bacteria that were trying to grow and reestablish themselves are washed out, leaving the field entirely to the fungus.

We women think we are being clean but actually we are causing problems by interfering with the natural environment and encouraging fungal growth. The normal balance of bacteria in the vagina is there to keep an acid pH level of four. If the pH tips to the alkaline side, fungus starts to move in. Many women believe that because vinegar is acid, douching with vinegar will preserve a pH of four, but they are not douching with vinegar; they are adding a little bit of vinegar to water, which has a pH of seven, and the result is not the same as preserving the natural pH of four.

The only way to get rid of fungal growth is with antifungal medications—but not over-the-counter preparations because they may encourage the emergence of different strains of fungus. Rather than trying to treat yourself, see your gynecologist. Better still, do not douche in the first place. If you have a malodorous discharge, again, see your gynecologist. Perhaps there is an overgrowth of a particular bacteria or perhaps you have picked up a venereal infection. Whatever it is, you will have a better chance of getting it remedied quickly than the woman who tries to deal with the discharge herself and waits a couple of months before seeking professional help. By that time the evidence is lost, and the gynecologist is doing culture after culture trying to identify the offending organism. On the other hand, walk into the gynecologist's office, say "I have this bad odor," and boom! there's your organism, that's it, we can take care of it. (See chapter 18.)

If women did not douche, I venture to say that it would save millions of dollars in gynecologic visits. Months of suboptimum treatment with home remedies so obscure what the original problem was that just about the best the doctor can do is to try one thing, and if that does not work, try another, and then a third and a fourth; and the poor patient has to keep coming back and back and back.

As well as the problem of an invasion of fungus, there is the possibility of causing pelvic inflammatory disease by douching. The vagina with its bacteria is separated from the uterus by the cervix, and the uterus is sterile. Use a douche and the bacteria safely in their hometown of the vagina may suddenly be picked up and flushed into the uterus, where they have no business being and where they can cause infection. The infection may damage the fallopian tubes and increase the chance of an ectopic pregnancy, "ectopic" meaning "out of the normal place."

Forget the folklore that says women have to run to the bathroom and douche every time they have intercourse. The vagina is open-ended and most of the semen drains out. When you stand up, it is out of there, and any remnant left behind is quickly whipped away by the bacteria in the vagina.

One of my female professors in medical school used to say this: "Do you douche your eyes? Do you douche your nose? Then why are you douching your vagina? The body has a way of taking care of the eyes and nose, and it has a way of taking care of the vagina, a natural way of renewal, of keeping everything balanced, of making sure that no offending organisms will cause problems. Interfere with the natural balance and you are asking for trouble. In short, the only thing that should go in a vagina is a penis, the only thing that should come out is a baby."

The single reason to douche is if a physician has identified the offending organism, determined that it can be eradicated by using Betadine, and has instructed the patient to douche medicinally. The drawback here is that the next time the patient has symptoms, she is likely to assume she knows what is wrong, get Betadine from the drugstore, and treat herself, only to develop persistent vaginitis because the organism has become resistant or a different organism is involved.

The same thing is happening with the treatment for fungus. Physicians prescribe Monistat cream, which is now available over the counter. Patients, when they have a recurrence of symptoms, treat themselves with the cream and because of overuse, strains of fungus not susceptible to Monistat are appearing. As it becomes more and more difficult to treat vaginitis successfully, it is even more imperative that douching be avoided because douching is likely to be the prime cause. Contrary to rumor, vaginal infections are not picked up from toilet seats. If any personal area is at risk from a toilet seat, it is the external vulva, not the internal vagina. The vulva can get lesions from picking up something on the seat, but bacteria need a warm, moist area to grow, and toilet seats, unless you knock somebody off real quick and take her place, are usually cold and inhospitable to bacteria.

Swimming pools may be warm and moist, but chlorinated water kills anything. Lakes are a bit more problematic; microorganisms or parasites in the water can get in the vagina, but the risk is not very great. As for baths, some water may enter the vagina, but the angle of the vagina is such that when you stand up, it flows out, and less water enters than in a douche because the walls of the vagina meet when it is empty.

Actually, baths are a good idea—that is, if they are solitary baths, not baths in a communal hot tub, which can indeed spread infection. If women took baths rather than showers, many of the problems they have in the perineal area—the region between the thighs—would be obviated. It is here, in the pubic hair and on the vulva, that perspiration and moisture can encourage the growth of fungus and bacteria. It is a pity that bidets have never become popular in this country. If women used bidets and/or took baths instead of showers, vaginal and vulvar irritations would occur considerably less often.

Douching to Prevent Pregnancy. The most emphatic thing that can be said about the use of douching to prevent conception is that it does not work. With the woman lying down, when the man ejaculates, the semen is deposited at the top of the vagina in a pool under the cervix, and with the woman's orgasm, the cervix dips down into the pool and siphons up the ejaculate. Even without orgasm, the semen can enter the cervix like seepage from a pond and travel from there to the uterus. If the woman gets up and douches, no matter how quick she is, the sperm are quicker. By the time she douches, it is already too late. The sperm are on their way.

There does not even have to be an ejaculate. In the clear fluid on the tip of the penis before ejaculation, several hundred sperm are present. Patients say to me, "We didn't do anything, Dr. Thornton. All we did is just that he was very close." I have to tell them, "That's all it takes. The little buggers go, 'Oh, vagina? Thanks!' and Bingo! you are pregnant." The ovum is fertilizable only for 24 hours, but sperm can last five to seven days in the vagina, hanging around waiting for that egg to come out. The fact of the matter is that we are made to have offspring. Mother Nature set it up that way. Egg and sperm are going to get together if they possibly can, and douching is unlikely to stand in their way.

At the opposite extreme, douching can impact upon a woman's fertility in the future. It may make it impossible for her to conceive because douching has moved bacteria where they have no business being and they have caused pelvic inflammatory disease. The fallopian tubes become infected, and their cilia, the lashlike processes as fine as hairs that propel the egg toward the uterus, become clublike. It is as though the cilia develop arthritis and are no longer able to undulate, and without their flowing ripple to move the egg along, pregnancy is not going to happen. At least, it is not going to happen by the normal route; fertility specialists can bypass the tubes and plant a fertilized egg directly in the uterus; although this procedure does not always lead to a successful pregnancy. (See chapter 7.)

PAINFUL INTERCOURSE

Lubrication. Intercourse, coitus, and pareunia, which comes from the Greek word for "bedfellow," all mean the same thing. Dyspareunia, then, is the medical term for painful intercourse. So that my patients remember it, I sometimes joke that dyspareunia is better than no pareunia at all. Dyspareunia can affect a woman at any age, from the start of her sexual life into her seventies and eighties. The more sexually active a woman is, the less likely she is to experience it, while it is most apt to occur in someone who has been widowed and has not had intercourse for an extended period of time. When a widow finally finds a gentleman who makes her heart beat a little faster and one thing leads to another, that is when I get the phone call: "Dr. Thornton, oh my goodness . . ."

The source of the problem is that her vagina is not well lubricated, for lubrication is the key to pleasurable intercourse. Lubrication can be either natural or artificial, or some of both—that is, with some artificial augmentation of the natural lubrication that comes from the two Bartholin glands on either side of the vaginal opening. Natural lubrication does not require any discussion because the body knows exactly what to do, but when the body is not secreting enough lubrication, then augmentation with a sterile lubricant is in order.

Vaseline should never, ever be used for lubrication during intercourse. I cannot put the point too strongly because it is a longstanding myth that petroleum jelly is the answer to lubrication. It is not. It is an occlusive substance. It suffocates the pores in the perineal area, preventing them from contributing any natural lubrication at all and simply making matters worse. What is needed is a water-soluble lubricant, such as Surgi-lube, Astroglide, or Replens, any one of which aids immeasurably in the ability to have nonpainful intercourse.

These newer lubricants are like *spinnbarkeit*, a naturally occurring mucus produced by the cervix at midcycle. Just before ovulation the cervical mucus becomes very thin and elastic. If a gynecologist wants to know whether a woman has ovulated yet, he or she picks up a little mucus on an instrument and spreads the instrument apart. If the mucus stretches and stretches and is seemingly infinitely elastic, ovulation has not occurred. If, on the contrary, it is thick and sticky, then ovulation has occurred. Like spinnbarkeit, the newer vaginal lubricants now on the market are elastic and slick, as slick as oil on a road, and women who have had a problem with insufficient lubrication love them.

Infection. Another source of dyspareunia can be infection, such as herpes, and what is termed nonspecific vaginitis or bacterial vaginitis. Identification and treatment of the responsible organism take care of the problem.

Age. A third possible cause is, simply, age. With age comes a thinning of the vaginal epithelium, and that leads to severe dyspareunia in some postmenopausal women. Treatment is an estrogen cream, applied vaginally, that builds up the vaginal wall. Because the estrogen in the cream is absorbed as rapidly as from a pill taken orally, women must also take progesterone in order to avoid an increased risk of uterine cancer. The progesterone may cause some spotting—a withdrawal bleed after the progesterone dosage is finished—but often it does not. In any event, the progesterone is needed so that the effect of estrogen on the uterus does not go unopposed. The exception is the woman who has had a hysterectomy; she can use just the cream as long and as often as she wishes.

If the woman has hot flashes or is at risk for osteoporosis, the gynecologist may prescribe oral medication that equally will build up the vaginal wall, but if the patient's only complaint is dyspareunia, the cream is the treatment of choice. She may use it for three to six months and then find she does not need it anymore, or she may use it every other day or once a week and finally stop it on her own. How long the effect lasts varies. One patient will be back where she started two months after stopping use of the cream, another in six months, and another may say, "Well, I used it seven or eight years ago, and I've never had a problem since."

POINTS TO REMEMBER

- Keep a menstrual calendar.
- The length of a cycle is calculated from the first day of a cycle, not the last.
- The midpoint of the cycle is when ovulation occurs, with the midpoint calculated from the first day of the last period.
- Irregular bleeding should be evaluated at once.
- Do not douche.
- Do not treat a vaginal infection with over-the-counter preparations.

2

A PAP SMEAR IS NOT A PELVIC EXAM

❧

No woman likes to go for a pelvic exam. You never hear, "Oh, boy, I just can't wait to visit my gynecologist!" And why should anyone look forward to it? The position is ignominious; you feel like a plucked chicken spread-eagled on the table. The instruments may be icy. The poking around can be painful. The experience may be humiliating and dehumanizing. I have been on both sides of the stirrups and I know.

The first time I went to a gynecologist, I was about to be married and there were many questions I wanted to ask. I chose a woman physician and assumed we would have a warm and useful chat in her office before she examined me. Instead, a nurse ordered me to disrobe and don a paper gown, which, despite my clutching fingers, billowed one way while I billowed another. Self-conscious and draft-ridden, I sat on the table in the examining room and waited. For two hours. Nobody bothered to come tell me that Dr. X was delayed, and when Dr. X herself finally rushed in, she barely spoke, just ordered me into the stirrups and inserted a poorly made plastic speculum that pinched, then rushed off again without giving me a chance to ask the questions I had come with.

When a woman has an experience like that, it is not surprising if she tells herself that as long as her internist does a Pap smear once a year, she can skip being seen by a gynecologist. But a Pap smear does not really substitute for a pelvic examination. Let me describe what I think a thorough gynecologic examination consists of so that you will understand why this is so and why you may want to change gynecologists, as I did, if the experience is not a comfortable one. Once you have the information, you will know better what to expect and what to ask for, and because you will understand why certain procedures are necessary, you may well find that you mind the whole experience a great deal less.

WHEN SHOULD A WOMAN START SEEING A GYNECOLOGIST?

The American College of Obstetricians and Gynecologists recommends that a woman should start seeing a gynecologist at 18 years of age or whenever she becomes sexually active, *whichever comes first.* Females who have not had sexual intercourse tend to believe that if the hymen has not been perforated, the gynecologist cannot do an examination, but that is not the case. The hymen is fenestrated—that is, there is an opening or several small openings that allow the menstrual flow to emerge—and this fenestration permits a small speculum to be introduced, a speculum being an instrument like a pair of tongs that is used to spread the walls of the vagina apart. Either a baby Pederson speculum or a nasal speculum can be used to allow the gynecologist to view the vagina and cervix.

Children. In years of examining pediatric patients brought to me because the mother or the referring doctor wanted a female gynecologist, I have never had a problem in, first, viewing the vagina and cervix and then gently introducing one finger to examine the small uterus and ovaries. A child as young as seven may be referred because she has had some irregular bleeding. Usually there is nothing wrong, or she may have a small polyp. A botryoid sarcoma, which looks like a cluster of grapes hanging in the vaginal canal, is a cancer of young women, but only very rarely is that found to be the cause of the irregular bleeding.

Another reason for the examination of a young child is when sexual abuse is suspected. This is an emotional sort of situation and great tact is required, but still, if care is exercised, the examination can be carried out without risk of adding to whatever trauma the child has experienced.

Sexual Assault. Young women who have been sexually molested or assaulted should seek immediate medical attention through a hospital emergency room or family planning clinic. This is not a time for reticence. You may need to have medication or antibiotics to protect your future ability to have children because the act may have resulted in a sexually transmitted disease that can destroy the fallopian tubes. You do not want your future life to suffer because of an incident you were not responsible for, so this is the time to overcome your natural hesitation and seek medical help. You do not have to divulge anything—the emotional and psychological concerns can be evaluated a little later—but prompt medical help is needed so that cultures can be taken to see if you have been exposed to any of the venereal diseases, and your HIV status needs to be checked.

Sexually Active Women. If you have made the decision to become sexually active, no matter what age you are, it is important that you protect yourself, for intercourse may cause a change in your previous state of health. There may be a cyst or an abnormality such as two cervices that requires medical attention. Unintended pregnancy is, of course, a concern, and if the partner has had previous sexual experience, infection is a possibility. A gynecologist who already knows you is in a better position to evaluate an acquired infection, just as she is in a better position to offer advice about birth control measures. Gynecologists understand the pressures girls experience to become sexually active, and they are nonjudgmental, interested only in ensuring their patients' health and well-being.

WHY ALL THESE QUESTIONS?

History Taking. In my own practice, if a patient of any age is someone I have not seen before, she is shown, fully dressed, into my office, not the examining room. I introduce myself and ask her, if I am in any doubt, how her name is pronounced and I write the pronunciation phonetically on her chart. I also write down what she wishes to be called: Miss Smith, Mrs. Smith, Joan, or Joanie—whatever her preference is—so that the office staff and the nurses will know how to address her. A longstanding paternalistic tradition in medicine allows women to be called by their first names while the doctor is addressed by title and last name. Many patients feel, justifiably, that this puts them in a one-down position and they resent it. On the other hand, some younger patients feel it is friendlier to be called by their first name. Either way, it should be the patient's choice because how you are addressed has the power to make you feel good about yourself or quite small and worthless.

The only time I myself have trouble letting it be her choice is when the patient is an elderly lady. One such patient insisted I call her Beth; I said, "I'm sorry, Miss Bender, but I just can't do it. Something inside won't let me, so, please, just humor me." On the other hand, if you would like to be called by your last name and you go to an office where they automatically use your given name, it can be difficult to get them to change without sounding rude or standoffish. When it happens to me, I say, "Excuse me, but I don't like my first name, so I'd be grateful if you'd call me Dr. Thornton or Mrs. McClelland." Actually, I love my first name, but it is the technique comedians use of saying something self-disparaging to disarm the audience before coming in with the zinger.

If the patient gives her name as, let us say, Patricia Sweeney, I inquire if Sweeney is her married name. If so, I ask for her maiden name because Mrs. Sweeney may well have been Miss Marconi, and I will know that, with her Italian heritage, I should be on the lookout for thalassemia, or the patient may have been Miss Levy and I should check for Tay-Sachs disease. Ethnicity and inborn errors of metabolism, like Tay-Sachs in people of Jewish heritage or sickle-cell anemia in people of African heritage, are often linked.

I then take the patient's history. Many doctors, to save time, have the patient fill out a questionnaire while she is in the waiting room, but I like to look at my patient, see how carefully or indifferently she is dressed, how well or ill she looks, how troubled or at ease, and I like to inquire further into some aspects of the history. For instance, if the patient's mother died of epilepsy, I want to know whether the mother had a lifetime of seizures or a few at the end of her life. If the patient's father died of liver disease, I want to know if he was a heavy drinker and whether the patient herself has a problem with alcohol

When the patient hesitates over an answer, I try to probe further. Since all the time we have been talking we have been developing a rapport, often the woman will say, "I didn't want to tell the nurse, but . . ." and deeper concerns emerge that she might not have found an opportunity to voice otherwise.

Taking a history is more than a matter of establishing facts; it is a way of getting to know the whole person and what may be important in her care and treatment. I was taught in medical school that ninety percent of taking care of a patient involves listening and a careful history. "If you listen," my professors said, "the patient will tell you what's wrong with her. If you don't really listen and just assume you know the answers, a lot of the time you're going to be wrong."

The Preliminaries. After the history-taking, I turn the patient over to a nurse, who gives her a paper cup for a urine specimen and asks her to empty her bladder. There are two reasons for this: If the bladder is full, palpating the uterus is like trying to feel a change purse through a balloon; and I want to know if there is protein, sugar, or blood in the urine. The doctor who just tells the patient to go to the bathroom is missing a lot of information. Something as simple as dipsticking the urine sample detects the presence of protein, for example, and because bacteria give off protein, that starts me to thinking whether this patient has an infection. Or I pick up the presence of sugar and become concerned about the possibility of diabetes; blood, and I think about the possibility of kidney disease.

After she empties her bladder, the patient disrobes completely and slips a cloth poncho over her head—not a paper gown that gaps or a cloth gown that opens down the back and cannot be kept closed. One size assuredly does not fit all, especially the full-figured woman, and I want my patients to keep their dignity intact and be as comfortable as possible. The poncho and the examining table sheet allow any part of the anatomy not being examined at the particular moment to remain discreetly covered. Because I want the atmosphere in the examining room to be pleasant and relaxed, in my office the walls are painted a warm rose color and are hung with flower paintings; classical music plays softly; and the stirrups are padded so that warm feet do not come in contact with cold metal.

THE PHYSICAL EXAMINATION

Starting at the Top. Rather than proceeding directly to the pelvic examination, I first go over the patient in a general way to make sure that her basic health is good. With the patient sitting on the table, I look at her eyes to see if there is any yellowing or if she looks pale. Next I check the nodes under the chin and above the collarbone to see if there is any enlargement, which can be a sign of lung cancer. This check is particularly important if the patient is a smoker, a fact I have established with the history. After that I examine the thyroid.

The thyroid is a very, very important gland to the female reproductive system. With hypothyroidism—a thyroid gland that is underactive—the patient may have problems with her periods; they may be very irregular or not come at all, and she may have difficulty becoming pregnant. With hyperthyroidism—the secretion of too much thyroid hormone—she may lose weight and not be able to sleep at night. If the thyroid is enlarged, she may have a goiter. Even though as a gynecologist I am not an internist, I have felt enough thyroid glands to know whether this particular gland is larger or smaller than normal and whether there is a lump on it.

Next I look at the patient's back to see if she has scoliosis—curvature of the spine. Some people may have had it for a long time without being aware of it, and now they are having difficulty breathing or problems with their hips. A quick look tells me whether the spine is straight.

While still examining her back, I say to the patient, "Tell me if this hurts," and I pound her on the back on both sides where the kidneys are. If the patient has the beginnings of a kidney or urinary tract infection, she cannot stand to be banged on her back. Ninety-nine out of a hundred patients do not mind being hit, but the hundredth one who says, "Wow, that hurts!" has an infection.

Once while I was pounding a patient's back I noticed a little black spot. She had freckles all over, but one freckle looked darker than the others. The patient was dismissive. "Oh, I've had that for years," she said.

"Maybe so," I said, "but it has an irregular margin and it looks to me like it's growing. Just for the heck of it, let me send you to a dermatologist to check it." She agreed—and she went; some patients say yes to a referral but never follow up on it. This patient and I were both very glad she had because the little black spot proved to be a malignant melanoma, a skin cancer.

Breast Examination. Next I ask the patient to lie down on the table and I check her breasts. While I am doing this, I ask how long it has been since she did a breast self-examination. Often she says, "Yes, I know I'm supposed to do it every month, but I get so busy with the kids," et cetera. So then I emphasize the importance of self-examination and go over the procedure with her (see chapter 3).

I examine the breasts for any lumps or thickenings, any difference in size or shape, and the nipples for any discharge. Because the tail of the breast goes underneath the armpit, I check that area, too. This check is important; if it is left out of the examination, the knowledgeable patient will say, "Doctor, would you check under the armpit for me, please?"

Abdomen. There is always a story behind a scar, and if any are visible on the abdomen, I want to hear when the operation was and what it was for. After that, I press down on the abdomen here and there to detect whether there is pain, and I take a stethoscope from my pocket to listen to the abdominal sounds, which can range from a gurgle to a timpanic boom worthy of the Philharmonic. As long as I have the stethoscope in hand, I also listen to the heart—but that is because it is in my nature to be thorough; it is not a regular or expected part of the gynecologic examination.

On each side of the groin there is a large artery, the femoral artery, which serves the lower extremities, and there are also the inguinal nodes where the female reproductive tract drains. If a node is enlarged, it is a red flag alerting me to be on the lookout for infection or malignancy. The femoral artery has a pulse, just like the radial pulse in the wrist, and I palpate it. If it feels turbulent, I begin to wonder about an obstruction somewhere. In one patient, who had mild high blood pressure, I could feel no femoral pulse at all. "Have you had any headaches lately or problems with muscle fatigue or pain in your legs?" I asked.

"Oh, my children give me a headache and I think I've been exercising too much."

"Perhaps that's all it is, but I think you should see a vascular surgeon just to be sure," I said. She did, and it turned out she had a coarctation of the aorta, a narrowing of the aorta in the chest so severe that only a scant amount of blood was getting down to her legs and feet. The vascular surgeon was surprised that the patient had been referred by a gynecologist, but, as I say, a good gynecologic examination is concerned with the patient's general health, not just the health of the reproductive system.

Pubic Area. In the pubic area I look to see if there are any little things crawling around. It sounds dreadful but it does happen. I looked at one patient and saw something glistening in her pubic hair. I said to myself, "No, I can't be seeing that." I looked again—closely. I said to the patient, "Have you had any problem with itching lately?"

"Yeah, Doc! Also, I didn't want to tell you this but I've had funny little black specks in my underwear."

"Have you been with anybody?"

"Like a one-night stand with a guy I met at a party, is that what you mean?"

I put on gloves, pulled a hair, and put it under the microscope, and there it was: *Phthirus pubis*, an ugly little six-legged creature. "I hate to tell you," I said, "but he gave you crab lice."

Antilice medication takes care of the problem—a one-shot deal and it is over; but first the problem has to be identified. The gynecologist is like a mother with her child; the mother only has to glance out of one eye to pick up that the child is coming down with a cold. By the same token, the gynecologist is so familiar with the usual look of things that one glance tells her when something is amiss.

The Pelvic Exam Proper. Only now does the patient put her feet in the stirrups, lie back, and assume the dreaded dorsal lithotomy position. But by now, because we have been chatting, because I have not come right at her with this invasive examination, the patient's anxiety level has gone down. She is comfortable with me and I am comfortable with her.

Since the last thing I want is for her to tense up again, I choose the speculum I will use with care. The speculum spreads the vagina for viewing of the walls and the cervix, and one size, again, definitely does not fit all. If the patient has had three or four children, the vagina can accommodate the traditional large Graves speculum. If, on the other hand, the patient is a lady in her seventies whose husband has been dead for twenty years, there is no way even a medium-sized speculum can be inserted, not with any comfort at least. In an internist's office usually only one size is available, but a gynecologist has an array of sizes. In the average patient, who may or may not have had a child, the narrower Pederson speculum can do everything the larger Graves speculum does while causing less discomfort. For the elderly lady, a baby Pederson is indicated, although when that is what I want the nurse to hand me, I ask for a debutante speculum because patients react better to the sound of "debutante" than "baby."

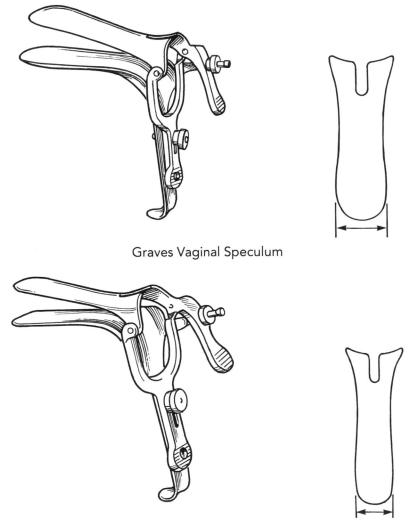

Graves Vaginal Speculum

Pederson Vaginal Speculum

Two Types of Specula

The nurse does not just reach back to a tray of instruments and pick up the speculum I have asked for. The room temperature is 72 degrees but the vaginal temperature is about 99 degrees; a metal speculum is going to feel like it is straight from the freezer and the patient will tense up, which, again, I do not want. Instead, the nurse takes the speculum from a bain-marie filled with warm water where it has been placed after being sterilized. The warm water is not sterile, but this does not matter because neither is the vagina; there are 23 types of bacteria there naturally, from *Bacteroides* to streptococcus to staphylococcus. As well as making the introduction of the speculum more comfortable, the warm water is an excellent source of lubrication, which is important because no jelly or other lubricant should be used on the speculum lest it interfere with interpretation of the Pap smear.

After collection of cells for the Pap smear comes visual inspection of the vagina. I look at the side walls to see if there are any lacerations, growths, herpes lesions, or whitish plaques. If I see anything out of the ordinary, I refer the patient to a gynecologist who specializes in colposcopy so that the area can be examined more closely and a sample collected to send to the laboratory.

I have already asked the patient, while taking the history, whether she is sexually active. When a doctor puts that question, she means *any* frequency or infrequency, but a patient may interpret it differently and say, "No, I'm not sexually active. I only have intercourse once a month," so I have to pin down what she means by her answer. If the patient has any sexual intercourse at all, I ask whether she and her partner are mutually monogamous, that is, whether either of them has sexual relations other than with the present partner. If she says they are not or that she cannot answer with certainty for her partner, I take a chlamydia culture. Sometimes when the patient gets the bill, she objects that she did not ask for this test. I explain that, "As your physician, I'm here to protect you from disease and infection, and chlamydia is a silent epidemic. You don't know you have it unless a culture identifies it. Probably the culture will come back negative, but if it doesn't, I'll need to treat you for the infection."

The Pap Smear. For the Pap smear (so called in honor of its developer, George N. Papanicolaou) it is necessary to collect samples of cells from the vagina, uterus, and cervix. First I scrape the outer surface of the cervix with an Ayre spatula, which looks like a wooden tongue depressor with an indented end. After smearing these cells on a slide, I place the indented end of the spatula against the cervix and sweep it around with the same gesture used to put on lipstick. Again the collected cells are placed on a slide and immediately fixed with fixative.

With the broader end of the spatula, I scrape cells from the vaginal wall to be examined for any indication of abnormality or infection. Because the cervix protrudes into the vagina, there may be some discharge underneath it, so cells are sometimes collected from there as well, but this is the least consequential part of the Pap smear and some doctors have done away with it in the interest of cost-effectiveness.

The third place for the collection of cells is within the cervix, in the endocervical canal. This is the really important part of the Pap smear because it is in this area that abnormal cells are most likely to begin their change toward malignancy. The canal is different in every woman. If the patient has never had a child, never been pregnant, and never had a termination of pregnancy, the orifice may be no larger than a pinhole, whereas if she has had three or four children, it will be somewhat dilated.

If it is dilated, even the nonspecialist in gynecology can insert a moistened Q-tip, rotate it, and collect endocervical cells to be spread on a slide. But if the cervical opening is not dilated and will not admit a Q-tip, the nonspecialist gives up at this point, calls the collecting done, and sends the slides off to the lab. The lab report comes back saying basically, "No endocervical cells seen, but the ectocervix is fine," and the doctor tells the patient her Pap smear was negative, meaning that all the cells examined were normal. But in reality the Pap smear was not negative; it was incomplete. A precancerous condition may be present within the cervix or uterus and go undetected because those cells were not collected.

The gynecologist, on the other hand, routinely uses an instrument called a cytobrush for endocervical sampling. The cytobrush looks like a miniature, collapsed Christmas tree. In the center of it is a very narrow filament, and folded back along this filament are tiny soft brushes like branches. The filament can be inserted through the smallest cervical opening. Once inside, the branches spread out, and when the cytobrush is twirled, an excellent sampling of endocervical cells is obtained.

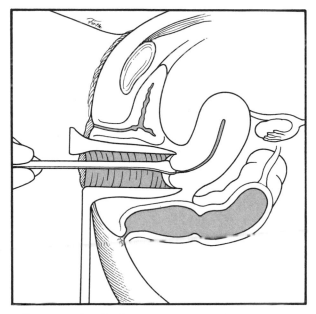

Collection of Cells for Pap Smear with Ayre Spatula

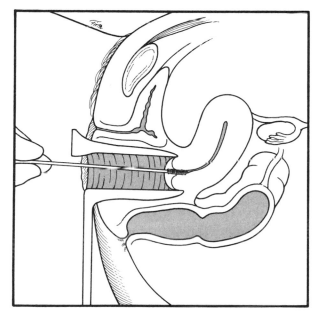

Collection of Cells from Inside the Uterus with Cytobrush

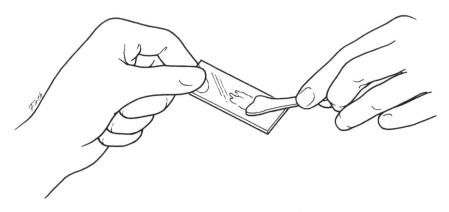

Cells Spread on Glass Slide

The cytobrush, which is fairly new, has been approved for use with everyone except pregnant women, in whom it has not been tested. Since it is easy to do the sampling with a moistened Q-tip in a pregnant cervix, it does not matter for these women, but it does matter for everyone else, and this is one of the reasons why the pelvic examination is best done by a gynecologist.

After a Pap smear there may be a slight amount of bleeding because tiny vessels and small capillaries have been disturbed in the collecting of cell samples to send to the laboratory. The bleeding will not be as heavy as a period, but there can be brownish staining or spotting, which is nothing to be concerned about. However, if it persists for more than a few days, it should be reported to the gynecologist.

Uterus and Ovaries. After the Pap smear comes the pelvic examination, which is one of the most difficult physical examinations to master. In the female anatomy the uterus is buried under the bladder and the large and small intestines. The bladder may be full. There may be fecal material going through the large intestine. The uterus may be tilted upward or backward. The ovaries lurk somewhere in the midst of the intestines and it can be like looking for a needle in a haystack to find them.

I confess that it was not until I graduated from medical school and had been a resident for three years that I was certain I was feeling an ovary. Before that, whenever my preceptor said, "Dr. Thornton, do you feel it?" I said, "Sure, yeah," because I didn't want the preceptor to think I was a dummy. The truth was I did not know what I was feeling, but I figured if the preceptor felt it, it was there and it was all right. There is a steep learning curve; your fingers have to get educated, and when finally mine did, it was like an epiphany. As a senior resident I was asked to do a consultation on a patient, and I was examining her when suddenly I said to myself, "Hey, wow, there's the ovary!" and from that moment on, I knew what an ovary felt like.

Now if I cannot feel an ovary and do not see a scar, which can be the case if the incision was a bikini cut and the scar is buried in the pubic hair, I say, "Mrs. Jones, have you had any surgery?"

"Oh, yes, I forgot to tell you that, Doctor."

"Did the surgeon take anything out?"

"Yeah, the left side, they took that out because I had an ovarian cyst."

I nod because now I am confident that if I cannot feel the ovary, it is not there. That kind of confidence is hard won. When I was a resident at Roosevelt Hospital in New York City, I often got calls from the internal medicine floor to come up and do a pelvic examination and I'd say, "Wait a minute, you're an internist and her uterus is no different than her heart or lungs. Why don't you do it?"

"Oh, no, we don't do pelvics," would be the hasty answer.

I remember one such call. The patient was a 65-year-old woman and her chart was a thick tome. She was anemic and she had had the "blue plate special": every known blood test, every cardiac and pulmonary function test—name it, and she had had it. Everything except a pelvic. "Pelvic deferred," the chart said. Again and again: "Pelvic deferred."

I examined her. "There's a mass here," I told the internist.

"There is? We didn't find it."

"You didn't find it because it's buried in the middle of the abdomen and you kept writing 'Pelvic deferred' instead of examining her."

I think of other examples, including a particularly sad one, a 23-year-old who died of an overwhelming infection from a pelvic abscess because the internists looked everywhere else for the cause of her 104-degree fever. Growing up, we are given strong messages about the private area of the genitals. Particularly as it concerns females, boys are warned not to touch and girls are trained not to allow touching, and these messages linger on in adults, even in doctors. This is something that women should be aware of so they can

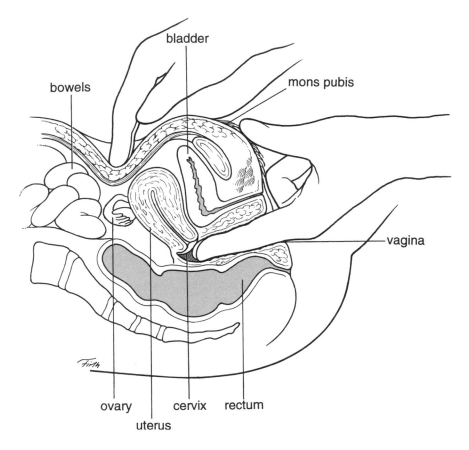

bladder

bowels

mons pubis

vagina

ovary   **cervix**   **rectum**

uterus

The Pelvic Examination

let their intelligence overrule their emotional reluctance to be examined and ask their doctors for a pelvic examination if they realize that area is being bypassed in the course of a medical workup.

To examine the pelvis, the gynecologist uses two fingers—the middle and index—of one hand, like a scout salute. The glove is lubricated and the two fingers are gently placed in the vagina. With the other hand the doctor presses down on the abdomen. With the bladder empty, the doctor can feel the uterus between her two hands and determine its size and shape and whether any lumps or bumps are present. Normally the uterus is tipped toward the front, but it can also be in the midposition, straight up, or tilted back toward the rectum.

Tilted Uterus. There are a lot of myths about a tilted uterus: that it prevents pregnancy, that it causes miscarriages, that it is the most common reason for reproductive problems in general. I used to believe these myths myself. I would see a woman in my practice with a severely retroverted uterus and say to myself, "Uh-oh, she'll probably never become pregnant" or, "Uh-oh, she's going to have one miscarriage after another." But after several years of having patients with tilted uteruses who had no problems at all, I searched the literature and discovered that a retroverted uterus is like being left-handed; it occurs in 10 to 15 percent of women and does not mean a thing.

When a woman is pregnant, as the fetus begins to grow, the uterus usually pops up by itself into the right position. In the very rare instances when it does not, it may have become trapped behind the bones of the pelvis; the doctor gives it a little push and that takes care of it. I cannot count the number of times I have been called on to examine a woman who is suspected of having a rectal tumor, only to have the mass prove to be nothing more than a retroverted uterus; it is that common.

Palpating the Ovaries. After examining the uterus, I palpate the ovaries. This is the point at which the examination can become uncomfortable because the ovaries in a female are homologous to the testicles in a male and no one needs to be told how a man feels about having his testicles squeezed. But it is important that the ovaries be palpated with enough pressure to determine how large they are and if there are cysts present.

Rectal Examination. At this point many doctors consider the examination over, but the uterus lies between the bladder and the rectum and what the doctor is examining through the vagina is merely the front side of the uterus. The posterior, or the back, of the uterus can not be accessed from the vagina, only from the rectum.

I ask the patient to bear down as though she is having a bowel movement. This dilates the rectum, and with extra lubricant I can insert a finger into it without discomfort to the patient and examine the back part of the uterus to make sure there are no masses or lumps. If I feel little irregularities on the supporting ligaments of the uterus, that raises my level of concern about endometriosis, a condition in which islands of endometrial tissue are found in abnormal locations outside the uterus.

When I withdraw my gloved finger, there may be a bit of fecal material on it, which makes this the ideal time to check for blood in the rectum by means of a hemoccult test. Blood can be an early sign of colon cancer.

Usually the test is negative but when it is not, I ask, "Mrs. Jones, have you been eating beets? Do you have hemorrhoids? Have you any history of rectal bleeding?" Depending on her answers, I have her repeat the hemoccult test at home. "I know it's disgusting," I say, "but it's important. From three different bowel movements, get a little bit of the stool, put it on the card, close the card up, and bring the packet back to the office, and I'll check it again. If it's still positive, I'll call you and give you the name of a gastroenterologist. It may be you have a polyp."

"Trying to get that specimen is like bobbing for apples," one patient said. So now I tell my patients, "Bob for the apple, get a specimen, and let's see if there's anything going on."

After the pelvic and rectal exam, there is one more thing: a look at the patient's legs and toes. The legs are the most common site of melanoma in women, and it takes only a moment to inspect them. Sometimes there are bruises, which may mean a blood clotting problem. The patient says, "I don't know, I seem to be bruising an awful lot lately," so then I do a complete blood count (CBC) and clotting studies. If the patient's platelets or clotting factors are low, I send her to a hematologist. If there are bruises but it does not look like a medical problem, I find an excuse to send the nurse out of the office, and I ask, "Has anyone been hurting you?" Statistics indicate 25 percent of pregnant women are battered; I see it often enough in my practice to believe it. The National Domestic Hotline is 1-800-799-7233.

TALKING IT OVER

Who Needs It? As long as it takes to describe this thorough gynecologic examination, the doing of it requires only ten minutes. Although the American Cancer Society recommends a Pap smear only once every three years if the previous three years have been negative, the American College of Obstetricians and Gynecologists advocates a yearly gynecologic examination because a lot can happen in three years and the chance may be missed to pick up a problem like an ovarian cyst in its early stages. When I explain this to my patients, they become conscientious about returning yearly, and often they decide their mothers should come in, too. Many a mother tells me truculently, "My daughter said I had to come here."

"I'm not here to hurt you," I say. "I'm here to help you. But if you truly do not want to be examined, I won't keep you. Tell me this first, though. How long has it been since you've seen a gynecologist?"

"Since Tommy was born. He's 26 now. But I've been okay, no problems, no pain or anything like that."

"Right, you haven't had any pain or bleeding or anything, so you're probably fine. But cancer is silent until it's at its end. That is when it causes pain, but then it's too late and you're up there with the angels."

"Well, if you put it that way . . ." Her brow furrows. "Are you sure cancer doesn't cause pain?"

"Not while it's making its way around and getting established. That's why I'm here—to put things on slides and send the slides to the laboratory so they can tell us everything is fine."

She hesitates. "Look, since my husband died, nothing's been in there."

"I understand. I'll be gentle."

"Well . . . okay, I guess you can go ahead." And that is the beginning of this lady's returning year after year because now she understands that it really truly matters.

The person who is hardest to convince that it matters is the woman who has had a hysterectomy. "It's out. No problem," she says. "I don't need a Pap smear." But there are different types of hysterectomies. One type just removes the top part of the uterus and leaves the cervix; another removes both the cervix and the uterus but leaves the ovaries; and a third removes uterus, tubes, and ovaries. A common misunderstanding among patients is that a total hysterectomy means the ovaries were removed, but that is not necessarily the case, and if any portion of the ovaries is still in place, that is a problematic area. If the cervix is still in place, cervical cancer, which kills almost 5,000 women each year, remains a possibility. Even if both ovaries and tubes have been removed along with the uterus and only the empty vault of the vagina remains, there can still be cancer of the vulva or vagina, which is infrequent but nasty.

All in all, there are quite sufficient reasons for a yearly Pap smear and pelvic examination—and quite sufficient reasons why they should be carried out by a specialist in gynecology rather than as part of a general medical checkup. There is an old joke about a gynecologist/obstetrician being no more than a catcher with a mitt and a wicker basket, that is, somebody to be there to catch the baby when it comes out, but I hope that by now you are persuaded that the gynecologist has a very large role to play in guarding your health and that the ten minutes you spend being examined by a gynecologist may be the most important minutes in your year.

POINTS TO REMEMBER

ON YOUR VISIT TO THE GYNECOLOGIST:
- Bring your menstrual calendar covering the previous six months.
- Know the *first* day of your last menstrual period.
- If married, give your maiden name as well.
- Make a list of all previous operations and all present medications.
- Tell your doctor if you bruise easily.
- On your initial visit, ask to be seen in the consulting room first rather than the examining room to allow some rapport to develop between you and the physician.
- Do not douche before the examination.
- A Pap smear can be done during your menses.
- Ask for the speculum to be warmed with hot water before the examination and for a Pederson speculum to be used if the examination is uncomfortable.
- Verify that a urine sample is tested for sugar and protein.
- Tell the doctor if someone is hurting you.

THE GYNECOLOGY EXAMINATION SHOULD INCLUDE:
- Examination of your neck and jaw to check pulses and for thyroid or lymph node enlargement.
- Breast examination should include the underarm area. Breast self-examination history and technique should be reviewed.
- The groin should be checked for pulses and enlarged nodes.
- The Pap smear should include an endocervical sample. The cytobrush is so far superior to the Q-tip applicator in obtaining an endocervical sample that if it is not used, you should ask why.
- A rectal exam is an absolute *must*, with the stool checked for blood (an early sign of cancer).

3

BREAST SELF-EXAMINATION

❧

SELF-EXAMINATION • TIMING • PROCEDURE • AN ASIDE ABOUT NIPPLES • FIBROCYSTIC BREAST DISEASE • MAM- MOGRAPHY • RISK • DISCOMFORT • MAMMOTHONS • TREATMENT •

Gynecologist-obstetricians see more breasts than any other doctor in any other specialty because all our patients are women. If we do not take advantage of this opportunity to convince patients about the importance of breast self-examination, we lose our best chance to eradicate advanced-stage breast cancer. Early detection, when the odds of curing the disease are high, is really up to women themselves.

What I tell my patients is this: You have to get to know your breasts as well as you know your face. If there was a blemish on your cheek, you would notice it immediately, and you have to be just that alert about your breasts and just that familiar with them. You have to look at them and examine them each month so that you are promptly aware of any change.

What we as gynecologists ask you as a patient to do is to notice a change. Come and tell us that what is there now is different from what was there before. Of course, if you never examine your breasts, you cannot do this. Women arrive at the gynecologist's office in a panic: "I have a lump in my breast!"

"Was it there before?" is the gynecologist's first question.

"I don't know. I've never examined my breasts. I've always been afraid of finding something."

That is the problem. Women are reluctant to examine their breasts because they are terrified of discovering a lump. They assume a lump means breast cancer, which it may well not, and they believe that if it is cancer, they will die of it, which they are unlikely to do if it is detected early. The lump does not care whether you are examining it or not, but if it is cancerous and is allowed to just sit there, its little cancer cells are multiplying: "Oh, thank you very much, we're here another month." By the time the lump is too apparent to be ignored and is causing skin changes, the cancer has gone to the lymph nodes and metastasized, and that is when the mortality rate climbs.

So, it is up to you to be vigilant—to say, "I am responsible for what God gave me, which means I am responsible for my breasts." Not your husband, not your boyfriend, not your doctor. I hear this: "My doctor examines them every time I have an appointment." How often is that? Once a year? Or: "My boyfriend examines them." Okay, is this your same boyfriend as when you last saw me? "No, he's the third or fourth." Or: "My husband examines my breasts." How often, after you have been married ten years, does a husband look at your breasts on a regular basis? None of this is good enough. *It is your responsibility.* They are your breasts. If you want to keep them, it is up to you to be completely familiar with their shape and feel.

Some women say, "I just don't want to touch myself." My answer is: "Come on, we have to be adult about this. You are a mother. You are a wife. People depend on you. You owe it to them to look after yourself. Eighty percent of masses are found by women themselves, not by doctors."

"That's what I'm afraid of—that I'll find something—and I'm too young to die."

"Sure, you're too young to die. But who says you're going to die? Eighty to ninety percent of all lumps are not cancerous."

"Really?"

"Yes! But if it does happen to be cancerous and you nip it in the bud, what do you think your chances are compared to the lady who either doesn't know the lump is there or does nothing in the hope that it will go away?"

"Better, I suppose."

"Much, *much* better."

There are women who acknowledge that self-examination is important but say, "Yeah, well, but do I have to do it every month?"

My stock answer is: "Only examine those breasts once a month that you want to keep. If you don't care whether or not you keep them, don't bother."

Then there are the women who go in for denial. They feel something but tell themselves, "It'll be okay." Why will it be okay? If it is, great. But if it is not, it should be caught early.

Doctors are adept at examining breasts because they do it over and over. But if you examine your breasts every month of your life, you become at least as much of an expert on them as the doctor who sees you once a year. Some breasts are pendulous; some are small. All have mammary tissue but mostly they are a conglomeration of fatty tissue, and it can be difficult for the doctor to be sure just what he or she is feeling. That is why a joint effort is needed. Your physician knows breasts, but you are the one who knows your own breasts and the two of you should work together as a team.

In the old days, if the woman said, "I have some sort of thickening here," and the doctor said, "Where? I can't feel it," the woman was likely to tell herself, "If he can't feel it, it must not be there." But now the woman who examines her breasts every month knows to be persistent and say, "It's a little thickening over here that wasn't there before. I know because I do an examination every month."

Let me tell you a personal story. I recently went for my gynecological exam, which I do yearly because I have two kids and I don't want to die. My gynecologist, a most meticulous man, said, "I think I feel something."

"What are you saying, you feel something?"

"When is your menstrual period?"

When I told him that I was at midcycle, I could see the relief on his face. Hormones are surging at midcycle and can cause breast engorgement, causing a difference in the feel of a breast. The doctor's confidence in attributing whatever he felt to this explanation was reinforced when I added, "I examine my breasts every month and I haven't felt anything, nothing that is any different from the way they always are."

The woman who does not examine her breasts cannot provide the doctor with this useful information. He feels something, she does not know if it was there before, and all of a sudden high anxiety sets in. She goes out of the office and gets hit by a bus because she is too panicked by the thought of breast cancer to look where she is going. On the other hand, if she does know her own breasts, she can say, "Look, Doc, I know you're good at what you do—delivering babies and hysterectomies and all that—but I know my breasts and I've had that little cyst for twelve years and it hasn't changed."

The habit of breast self-examination should be like brushing your teeth, just as much a part of your routine as that, and it should be started at a young age and continued as long as you live. Unlike that of other cancers, the incidence of breast cancer continues to rise with age. The peak incidence of cervical cancer is in a woman's 40s, of endometrial cancer in the late 40s and 50s, and of ovarian cancer in the 50s and 60s. But every time you add another candle to your birthday cake, you become more vulnerable to breast cancer, even at age 85.

The most recent statistics on breast cancer indicate that one in nine women will contract the disease. Breast cancer is the most frequent nongynecologic cancer in women, accounting for 32 percent of all cancers in women, and it is the second leading cause of death in women, exceeded only by lung cancer, which is less frequent but carries a higher mortality rate. Lung cancer is diagnosed at the rate of 72,000 new cases a year, with 59,000 women dying of it—a mortality rate of 81 percent—while 180,000 new cases of breast cancer are diagnosed each year, but with a morality rate of 46,000 or 25 percent. It may sound melodramatic to say that you can save your own life by establishing a routine of monthly breast self-examination, but it is no exaggeration.

SELF-EXAMINATION

Timing. Premenopausal women should examine their breasts at the time of the month when hormonal influence is at its lowest, that is, just after a menstrual period. We used to give instructions like, "When your period starts, count ten days" or "Wait until your period ends and count three days" or "Five days after the end of your period," but such dates are all too easy to lose track of and women were inclined to throw up their hands and do nothing. So now we couple the timing with something that women are aware of, which is the last day of the period. When a period tapers off, that is when you examine your breasts.

As an extra aid to remembering, put "BSE," for breast self-examination, on your menstrual calendar. For example, if your period started on the 10th of the month, when you mark that on your calendar, at the same time write BSE on the 17th so that you remember to do it. Don't do the examination before or during a period because the breasts may be tender and enlarged, making it difficult to know what you are feeling.

For postmenopausal women or women who have had hysterectomies and are no longer menstruating, the date to couple the examination with is the first of the month. As the months change, that is when you examine your breasts: "Ah, first of October, new month, got to examine my breasts."

Procedure. While you are waiting for the shower water to run hot, look at your breasts in the bathroom mirror to check that they are symmetrical, that one is not larger than the other, that neither is lopsided, and that the nipples are at the same level. God made us symmetrical, and if you notice any asymmetry, if you say to yourself, "Hm-m-m, they just don't look right," it can be a sign of disease— unless, that is, you have always been aware of some asymmetry and there is no change. *Change* is what you are most interested in.

Next look at the skin, whether there is any discoloration or dimpling or pitting. What we call *peau d'orange* is when pitting of the skin makes it look like the skin of an orange. Put your hands on your waist, elbows out, and lean over, and again look in the mirror for any pitting or dimpling.

After that, raise your arms above your head. If that has always been a perfectly smooth gesture but now something retracts, as though the skin is caught on something, that is to be noted and reported to your physician.

Now the water is hot and you get in the shower. Soap your body and before rinsing the soap off, examine your breasts by feel. Put one hand behind your head and with three fingers of the other hand make the Girl Scout pledge, crooking the little finger and holding it down with your thumb. Using the most sensitive part of your three fingers, which are the pads on the tips, go over the entire breast, making smaller and smaller concentric circles. When you get to the nipple, or what is called the areola, the darkened part of the breast, squeeze the nipple. Be gentle but put enough pressure on it to see if anything comes out. If there is a greenish discharge or if milk comes out and you are not lactating, give your doctor a call.

If you cannot be sure there is no discharge because of the soap, rinse the nipple off sufficiently to be able to see. The areolar part of the nipple may have little hairs growing out of it, which is normal, as are little glands—Montgomery glands—in the darkened part. The concern is to make sure there is nothing under the areola both by feel and by checking for discharge.

Before going through the same procedure on the opposite side, run your fingers up into your armpit and check for any thickening there in the tail end of the breast. Do both sides, rinse, finish your shower, dry off, and put lotion or baby oil on your skin. Then lie down on your back on a bed. Place a pillow under the side you intend to examine to move the breast toward the center. Now, do the same thing you did in the shower: the concentric circles, squeezing the nipples, checking the armpit. The difference now is that the breasts are on the chest wall and can be felt in relation to the wall.

So there it is, breast self-examination: simple, requiring only ten minutes once a month, indispensable, life-saving.

An Aside about Nipples. The reason for examining the armpits is because breast tissue extends that far. When we are embryos in our mother's womb, we actually have nipples that start from the armpit and go all the way down to the groin. These nipples undergo atresia—disappearing and leaving behind only the two nipples we traditionally see. But it can happen through a developmental hitch that some nipple tissue may persist, visible as little discolorations on the side of the belly or in the armpits, or there can be another nipple under the regular one or in the armpit, along with a bit of breast tissue.

It is worth describing this phenomenon because after a woman delivers a baby and starts lactating, she may have this udder in her armpit and think, "Oh, my God, I just had a baby and now I've got cancer." Not true. Nothing to get excited about. Most likely it is just an accessory nipple and accessory breast tissue, and as soon as lactation ends, it will disappear. But just to be on the safe side, see your doctor.

I have had patients deliver a baby and then have to go to the intensive care unit because of a complication like high blood pressure. The nurses and doctors in the ICU are not used to seeing postpartum patients, and when they detect this swelling under the patient's arm, I get a call: "Quick, quick, something's wrong. It could be malignant." But it is not, of course. It is mammary tissue reacting to another pituitary hormone, prolactin, the hormone responsible for lactation.

I should add, however, that if you are prepubertal or post-menopausal, the likelihood of its being mammary tissue reacting to prolactin is basically nonexistent, so if you feel a swelling or growth in the armpit, you should see your doctor.

FIBROCYSTIC BREAST DISEASE

Fibrocystic breast disease is cysts of the breast that are surrounded by tough, fibrous tissue, making the breasts feel lumpy, particularly during menstruation. For two reasons, it is important for women with this condition to know their own breasts. First, some women become emotional cripples because of constant worry that the lumps mean breast cancer, and they need to become so familiar with what is "normal" for them that they are not panicked by the discovery of a lump. Second, sometimes a cancer may be hidden behind a cyst, and if the woman does not know where the cysts are and is not familiar with their size and shape, she misses a chance to detect the change.

When I urge breast self-examination on women with fibrocystic breasts, they tend to say it is useless because they have lumps all over the place, but I insist that that is no excuse. Touch can be exceedingly acute when it is sensitized to the feel of things. Imagine, for instance, that you are left blindfolded in the desert. At first, you will not know one rock from another, one gully from another, but in just a short time of feeling your way about, you will be able to orient yourself perfectly by the slight differences between one rock and another, one gully and another. In the same fashion, you must become geographically expert about your breasts. You have to get to know each lump, where it is located, whether it is getting larger or smaller, whether it was there the month before or not. The important thing, just as with normal breasts, is change. If you detect a new lump, it probably just means you have developed another cyst, but still the mass needs to be diagnosed.

Many women believe that having fibrocystic breast disease increases their risk of cancer, but that is not true. It is a benign situation. The only risk is that the lumpiness of the breasts may allow a cancer to grow undetected. To obviate this possibility, a woman with a history of fibrocystic disease should be on very good terms with her breasts and with her breast specialist.

As for treatment of fibrocystic breast disease, there is none that is consistently efficacious. If somebody could come up with a drug treatment, he or she would become a millionaire overnight because the condition makes many women miserable. In the meantime, the best suggestion I can make to my patients is to try vitamin E—400 international units once or twice a day—which seems to help some patients. Vitamin B₆ is also sometimes recommended. If one of these works to relieve the aching, so much the better.

MAMMOGRAPHY

Mammography is examination of the breasts by means of X-rays. How often a woman should have a mammogram is a matter of some dispute between the National Cancer Institute and the American Cancer Society. Initially, they both agreed that a mammogram at age 35 to provide a baseline should be followed by another at age 40 and one every two years after that until age 50, then annually from age 50 on. A few years ago, however, the National Cancer Institute changed its recommendation to no mammograms at all between ages 40 and 50 and annually after age 50.

The American College of Obstetricians and Gynecologists, comprised of physicians who see patients and have to make recommendations, sides with the American Cancer Society: a baseline at age 35 for high-risk patients, then every one to two years from ages 40 to 49, and one every year from age 50 on. In a woman with a history of cystic breast disease, a mammogram should be done even more often. The screening of women by means of mammography is credited with increasing the five-year survival rate in localized breast cancer from 78 percent in the 1940s to 93 percent in 1993.

I was in my 40s when the National Cancer Institute withdrew its recommendation for a mammogram every two years between ages 40 and 50. Being no more eager than any other woman to have a mammogram, I said to myself, "Why should I go to the radiologist when the National Cancer Institute says I don't have to?" I let three years go by, until suddenly I asked myself, "Am I crazy? I'm the one who's going to get the breast cancer. They can withdraw their recommendation if they want, but these are my breasts and I want to keep them so I'm going back to regular monitoring." I would recommend to every woman that she do the same.

Risk. Many years ago there was a concern that mammography itself might cause cancer because of the radiation emitted during the procedure. But with the introduction of low-dose mammography, the amount of radiation involved is less than the radiation absorbed from the atmosphere if you take a plane from California to New York or climb a high mountain. In short, the radiation involved in mammography has been demonstrated not to increase a woman's risk of developing cancer.

Discomfort. Mammography should be done right after a period, not just before or at midcycle. There are two reasons for this. One is pain. Premenstrually, there is more fluid in the whole body. You are bloated, and with the breasts fuller and more tender, it is no pleasure to have them compressed, pressed down to about an inch thickness like flapjacks on a griddle. The more compression there is, the better the view the radiologist has, but it cannot be denied that it is uncomfortable. The second reason the mammography should be scheduled for the last day of a period or shortly thereafter is that some women have cystic changes in their breasts prior to the onset of their menses and this can confuse the mammography results.

Mammothons. While you are in the radiologist's office, look around the walls for a certificate of accreditation by the American College of Radiologists. This accreditation means that the radiologist is well qualified to interpret the X-rays. By the same token, be leery of mammothons—mobile mammography at a health fair. The intent is noble but the execution is usually flawed because there is no radiologist in the van. The customary procedure in mammography is for the patient to be asked to wait while the radiologist reviews the films so that, if the angle is poor or additional views are needed, more films can be taken immediately. If the screening is being done in a van and the van has to move on to the next neighborhood, that opportunity is lost.

Two things are important in mammography: the expertise of the technician taking the mammogram and the expertise of the radiologist interpreting the mammogram. They go hand in hand. With a poor technician there will be a poor scan that cannot be interpreted by the best radiologist. On the other hand, the technician can be first-rate, but if the radiologist is not Board-Certified and has not reviewed countless mammograms, he or she is going to miss things that should be caught. My own preference is to refer patients to a facility that is well versed in mammography rather than send them to a radiologist who does the procedure infrequently. As in all of life, experience tells.

TREATMENT

If I and/or the patient have detected a change in a breast and a suspicious area appears on the mammogram, what then? I do not believe a gynecologist-obstetrician should try to aspirate the lump to determine whether or not is a cyst (cysts have liquid centers, while tumors are solid); cells can be seeded along the route of the needle used to try to withdraw fluid from the lump unless the physician knows the area and the procedure very, very well. I refer the patient to a breast specialist—actually, a breast surgeon but I do not say "surgeon" because the word is so emotionally charged.

Some patients run for the hills if they hear the word *surgeon*. Immediately they envision their breast in a jar in the laboratory, and they do not follow through on the referral. Instead, they deny, deny, deny. When I was first in practice, I said "breast surgeon" to a patient. The following year I remarked that I hadn't received a report from the breast surgeon I sent her to. The patient started to cry and admitted she had never gone because she was afraid of surgery.

"Those breast cells are not crying," I told her, feeling nodes that had not been there the year before. "They've been having a happy time multiplying." Fortunately, with treatment, the patient survived, but the experience made me wonder what I could best tell women that would not strike fear into their hearts. I was sending them for a consultation to, yes, a surgeon, but to someone who was a breast specialist, so that was how I phrased my referrals from then on.

Depending on the clinical picture, the breast specialist may first try needle aspiration of fluid from the cyst. Any fluid withdrawn is sent to a laboratory for analysis. If fluid cannot be withdrawn because the lump is solid, the next step is more intensive mammography or an ultrasound examination of the breast and a biopsy.

Biopsy establishes whether the lump is a fibroadenoma—a solid tumor very common in young women and easily plucked out, rather like shelling a pea. Fibroadenomas are benign. If the diagnosis links "adeno" with sarcoma or carcinoma, as in fibroadenosarcoma or fibroadenocarcinoma, then the tumor is the malignant form. If the fibroadenoma is very small and in a young woman, the breast specialist may decide it can be left in place, but in an older woman the decision is almost invariably to take it out.

In the old days, if a frozen section done at the time of biopsy revealed a malignancy, the procedure continued on to major surgery, but now surgeons wait for a full biopsy report and make recommendations based on that—perhaps for a lumpectomy (segmental resection), perhaps for breast removal alone, perhaps for breast removal with reconstructive surgery. The surgeon will call me and say, "I haven't told the patient yet, but I will, so I'm going to tell you ahead of time what I will be saying to her in case she is upset and calls wanting input from you." He does not ask my advice about the treatment he proposes, nor should he because he is the expert in this area, not I. If the patient calls, I listen and talk things over with her but I do not make any recommendation. I think it is important for doctors to be honest about their limitations. Give me a baby to deliver or a hysterectomy to perform, fine; I am trained in those areas. But what training have I had in thoracic surgery? Like 99 percent of gynecologist-obstetricians, none. So I defer to people who are qualified and who know the protocols that have been established with regard to treatment of breast cancer.

The one bit of advice I have to pass on is the following. You may love your obstetrician. You have been going to him or her for years. He or she has delivered your babies. You have faith in him or her. All to the good. But when the problem is a breast problem, go to a breast specialist. Get it taken care of in the most expeditious manner possible by someone who knows how to handle the problem with the best chance of success. If you are my patient, this means not that I am abandoning you but, rather, that I am entrusting your care to someone with more expertise than I have, while still being there for you and still being kept in touch with the situation by the specialist.

POINTS TO REMEMBER

- Nothing is more important to your health than monthly breast self-examination. Eighty percent of breast cancers are found by patients themselves.

- Examine your breasts on the last day of your menstrual period when hormonal influence is at its lowest. Write "BSE" on your menstrual calendar as a reminder.
- For nonmenstruating women, the first of each month is an easy date to remember.
- What you are looking for is change, for something that is different from the way it looked or felt the previous month.
- Report to your physician any change you detect in the size, shape, or feel of your breasts or in the skin overlying them.
- Having fibrocystic breast disease is no excuse not to do breast self-examination. It is particularly important for the woman with lumpy breasts to become an expert in the size and location of cysts so that she can quickly detect any change.
- If you have a history of breast problems, you and your breasts and the breast specialist should be on very good terms and get together frequently.
- Have a baseline mammography at age 35; from 40 to 49, have one every two years; after 50, have one every year.
- Ask to be referred to a Board-Certified radiologist.

4

CONTRACEPTIVES: THE CHOICES

❧

THE PILL • SIDE-EFFECTS • DEPO-PROVERA • NORPLANT • THE DIAPHRAGM • THE CERVICAL CAP • THE MALE CONDOM • THE FEMALE CONDOM • THE IUD • STERILIZATION • RHYTHM METHOD • EMERGENCY CONTRACEPTION •

According to the National Center for Health Statistics, the most common form of contraception in use today (30%) is sterilization, that is, bilateral tubal ligation in the female or vasectomy in the male. Of this 30 percent, 18 percent is female sterilization, 12 percent male. Birth control pills are the second most popular form of contraception. Almost 10 million women use the Pill, making it responsible for 17 percent of contraception. Thus, the Pill and sterilization together account for almost half of all contraceptive methods in use.

In third place in popularity is the condom, accounting for 11 percent of contraceptive usage. This is the condom as used by the male; no statistics are available for the female condom, which, as far as I am aware, has not really gained much acceptance. The diaphragm is fourth in popularity. After that come IUDs, coitus interruptus, and periodic abstinence or the rhythm method. For those unfamiliar with the term "coitus interruptus," it is the practice of interrupting intercourse prior to ejaculation, sometimes referred to as "withdrawal"; since sperm are present even before ejaculation, the failure rate of this method of contraception is relatively high.

Of the 57.9 million women of reproductive age in the United States, roughly 40 percent use no form of contraception. Of these, 15 percent are not at risk of pregnancy, either because they are already pregnant, they are trying to become pregnant, or they have been sterilized. This leaves, at rough estimate, four million women between the ages of 15 to 44 having unprotected intercourse—unprotected meaning no birth control pill, no condom, no rhythm method. Obviously, this accounts for a lot of unintended pregnancies, particularly among teenagers.

Girls say, "It's not going to happen to me," and then it does—more frequently to African-Americans than to whites. For example, pregnancy rates in Alabama in 1991 were 139 per thousand black teenagers versus 77 per thousand white teenagers. In New York the figures were 173 per thousand in blacks, 76 per thousand in whites. Why, and why ours is a bicultural society, are social questions I cannot answer. I only know that the number of unintended pregnancies is appalling—black or white.

The fact of the matter is that Mother Nature considers us to be in this world to have children. Woman, the female of the species homo sapiens, is here to procreate, to go forth and be fruitful. Mother Nature does not care if you have completed your education, if you intend to be, or already are, an architect, a lawyer, a dentist, or a physician. As far as she is concerned, you are here to make certain that the human race continues, that it does not go the way of the dinosaurs. Crossing your fingers and saying, "Oh, I won't get pregnant this once," does not work—not for long, anyway.

The odds of avoiding unintended pregnancy are much better if some form of contraception is used, but none of the contraceptives is infallible. Each method has its failure rate. The average failure rate with birth control pills is 6 percent. This is not the fault of the Pill—if used perfectly, the failure rate is 0.1 percent—but women say, "I'm going on a weekend with my honey. Oh, dear, I left my pills home in the bathroom. I guess I'll just have to take a chance." The rhythm method, or periodic abstinence, has a 24 percent failure rate. Spermicides have a 30 percent failure rate. The condom and the diaphragm each have a failure rate of 16 to 18 percent. Even sterilization has a 3 to 4 per thousand failure rate. Mother Nature is not kidding. She is saying, "I don't care what you're devising down there, you are going to become pregnant." Riskiest of all, of course, is trusting to luck; using no contraceptive method has an 85 percent failure rate.

TABLE 1.

Contraceptive Failure Rates*

Method	Perfect use	Average use
No method (chance)	85.0	85.0
Spermicides	3.0	30.0
Withdrawal (coitus interruptus)	4.0	24.0
Periodic abstinence	9.0	19.0
Cervical cap	6.0	18.0
Diaphragm	6.0	18.0
Condom	2.0	16.0
Pill	0.1	6.0
IUD	0.8	4.0
Tubal sterilization	0.2	0.5
Injectables	0.3	0.4
Vasectomy	0.1	0.2
Implants	0.04	0.05

*Estimated percentage of women experiencing an unintended pregnancy in the first year of use.

Source: The Alan Guttmacher Institute. Facts in Brief: Contraceptive Use. New York: 1992.

THE PILL

Enovid, the first birth control pill, was introduced in 1960. The woman was to take one pill a day for 21 days and then have seven days with no pill, which would bring on her period. But because women often forgot to restart the pill regimen after seven days and consequently became pregnant, the majority of manufacturers now supply 28 pills, 21 of which are active and seven are placebos. This 28-day cycle, with one pill taken each and every day, keeps women on track and has cut down the failure rate.

The pills contain estrogen and progestin, a synthetic progesterone. The two hormones work together to suppress ovulation. It is as if you were pregnant; the two hormones put the ovaries to sleep, just as they do naturally when you are pregnant. They do this for 21 days. On the twenty-first day, you take the last active pill, and three days later your period comes. Your body says, "Okay, where are the hormones?" and when they do not appear in the bloodstream, your body responds by shedding the endometrial lining, resulting in menstrual bleeding.

The pills keep a sustained level of estrogen and progesterone in the bloodstream. A sudden fall in this level affects the endometrial lining, which is why spotting can occur if you forget to take the Pill. Patients come to me with the complaint: "I'm taking the Pill and I'm spotting." My first question is always whether they missed a day of the Pill; the answer is usually, "Oh, yeah, I forgot it one day." Incidentally, if you miss two days, forget about the Pill's contraceptive powers until the start of the next cycle; use some other contraceptive method or abstain in the meantime.

The pill should be taken *at the same time every day*, not in the morning one day and in the evening the next. The best approach is to link the pill-taking to an activity you do routinely, such as brushing your teeth or taking a shower.

The prevailing, but inaccurate, understanding is that you have to take the birth control pills for a month initially before you are protected from unintended pregnancy. Actually, you are protected after seven days. With the newest form of the pills you start taking them on the first day of your period; after seven days your period will have finished, and since women do not usually have intercourse during their flow, protection has been instituted by the time it is needed.

Side-Effects. In the early years of the Pill's introduction, thrombophlebitis—a painful swelling commonly called milk leg—was a concern, but this occurred because there was uncertainty about the hormonal dosage needed to suppress ovulation. When oral contraceptives were first approved by the Food and Drug Administration (FDA) in 1960, most Pills contained 150 micrograms of estrogen and 10 milligrams of progestin. Now the amounts have been reduced to 35 micrograms of estrogen and less than one milligram of progestin, and with these dramatically reduced dosages, side-effects have become rare. The package insert still gives a laundry list of everything that can happen or has happened at any time anywhere in the world to any woman, but this is because the pharmaceutical companies are protecting themselves from liability and should not be a cause for concern as long as the Pill has been prescribed appropriately and not "borrowed" from a girlfriend.

One of the things that women themselves are inclined to blame on the Pill is weight gain. Putting on pounds can happen but it is uncommon, unlike the old days when the large dosages of hormones led to fluid retention and weight gain. Now the hormonal amounts are so small that the Pill should not affect anyone's ability to gain or lose weight. What it can affect is the woman's mind; like the excuse of pregnancy, many a woman uses it to free herself from guilt about overeating. (See chapter 5 for a method of determining your ideal weight.)

A strong warning: *Never smoke while you are taking the Pill.* There is a statistically significant increase in heart attacks, strokes, and death in women who smoke while they are on the Pill. No one really knows why this is so. What I do know, though, is that I have seen too many young women with strokes in the intensive care unit.

One young woman was a patient of mine and the neurologist came to me saying, "I just don't understand it, she's only 24 years old and she's not on the Pill."

"Yes, she is," I said. "But she doesn't want her mother to know. That's why she denies it."

Smoking cigarettes and taking the Pill are both activities you have a choice about. You do not have to be on the Pill and you do not have to smoke. But if you are going to do one, do not engage in the other. This holds true for not just young women but women of any age; indeed, the older the woman, the greater the risk. I state the case as forcefully as I can to my patients, and if they still insist they want to be on the Pill but intend to continue smoking, I make them sign a disclaimer: "I have been informed by Doctor Thornton about the risks of smoking in combination with use of oral contraception. Nevertheless, I choose to use oral contraception."

"I can't stop smoking," the woman says. "I've tried and tried and tried."

"Then why not use a diaphragm?"

"No, I don't want to."

"Well, you're going to die."

"I don't care. I'll take my chances."

"Sign right here."

Having said all that, it is time for a good word about the Pill. It has liberated women. They are no longer shackled to unintended pregnancies. Plus, far from causing cancer, as has sometimes been rumored, the Pill actually helps to protect women against ovarian cancer, the cancer that is the greatest killer of women. It also lowers the risk of endometrial cancer. This protection does not require ten or twelve years on the Pill; if you have been on the Pill for two or three years, your risk for either of these cancers is lower than for women who have never used oral contraception, and that lowered risk continues indefinitely even if oral contraception is discontinued.

All in all, the Pill is still the best form of reversible contraception that does not involve any invasive measures, as do Norplant and Depo-Provera.

DEPO-PROVERA

Unlike the Pill, which contains both estrogen and progesterone, Depo-Provera contains only progesterone. The progesterone suppresses ovulation, thickening cervical mucus and altering the lining of the womb, thus preventing pregnancy and in many cases eliminating the shedding of the lining, that is, menstruation. Depo-Provera (medroxyprogesterone acetate) is in sustained release form and is given by injection in the buttock every three months. The injection is customarily carried out by a physician or a nurse practitioner rather than self-administered because it is a large dose of medication that has to be given at the proper site to avoid needle abscesses. Inadvertently injected into the sciatic nerve, for example, it can cause real trouble.

Depo-Provera, widely used in Latin America because it is so much cheaper than the Pill, is effective and safe, and its effects are reversible; if you want to get pregnant, you simply stop taking it. On the downside, in addition to the necessity of injections, some women experience irregular bleeding; they spot and spot and spot, which becomes such a problem that they have to get off the Depo-Provera. The majority of women on Depo-Provera have no periods, which they may well consider a blessing, but equally they have no way of knowing if they are pregnant. Having a period is a signal that the uterine lining is not being used as a succulent carpet for a growing embryo. Without that signal, a pregnancy test every two or three months is necessary.

NORPLANT

The Norplant system of contraception consists of six matchstick-sized silicone capsules of progesterone implanted one by one in a fan shape under the skin of the woman's inner arm, where slowly they degrade and provide highly effective contraceptive protection for five years. The failure rate with Norplant is an impressively low 0.05 percent.

However, again, there are drawbacks. After five years the capsules must be surgically removed. If the body has encapsulated these foreign bodies, surrounding them with fibrous tissue, or if they have migrated deeper into the tissues, they can be hard to locate. The supposed five minute removal time may stretch to an hour or more, and the tunneling down in search of the capsules can cause considerable pain, bleeding, and scarring, especially in women of color, who have an increased incidence of keloid formation from any sort of trauma.

In addition to the possible problems involved with removal, Norplant has been associated with an increased incidence of ectopic pregnancy and bleeding irregularities. About one in five women experience headaches, sometimes severe, that are initiated by the implants but are not necessarily ended by their removal. The same is true of hair loss; there may be a noticeable loss of scalp hair during the first year, and there is no assurance that it will be reversed by removal of the Norplant. Other concerns are numbness, tingling, and arm pain associated with the implantation process. Finally, there is an increased risk of myocardial infarction, or heart attack, as there is with all types of hormonally based contraceptive medication.

The market for contraceptives is, of course, huge, so there is a lot of salesmanship involved. For Norplant, the marketing went like this: "Why bother with the Pill when with just a little incision these six matchstick-sized capsules of progesterone can be implanted and for five years you have no worry about getting pregnant?" But the spiel was one thing, the reality another. These implants are often inserted by health care providers without surgical training who learn the technique from videotapes provided by the manufacturer. That little incision can cause scarring, and when the five years are up, the attempt to remove the matchsticks may result in downright disfigurement.

A woman who can afford the Pill is probably not going to want to have her arm cut. But if the woman is poor or is a sometimes irresponsible teenager or is socially or economically disadvantaged, Norplant is a very useful form of contraception. Birth control clinics may recommend it for women who cannot afford or do not have access to birth control pills or IUDs, and Medicaid will pay the five- or six-hundred-dollar cost.

THE DIAPHRAGM

The diaphragm is one of the oldest, most reliable forms of barrier method ever devised—*barrier* meaning a device that prevents the sperm from entering the uterus. I am sure that if your grandmother or mother was not careful enough, you saw a diaphragm in her bathroom when you were a kid. I know I did and wondered what that little dome-shaped rubber thing was.

That little rubber dome has prevented a host of unintended pregnancies (it is no longer politically correct to speak of "unwanted" pregnancies). But the diaphragm in and of itself is worthless. If after being fitted at your gynecologist's office, you buy and pay for the diaphragm at the pharmacy, take it home, and put it in but forget to place spermicidal jelly inside the cap, you may say, like some women who have come to me, "I used the diaphragm you prescribed. How come I'm pregnant?"

"Tell me how you used it," I say. "Did you listen to the instructions I gave you?"

"Sure. I put it in. It fit."

"What about the jelly?"

"What jelly?"

And there is the answer to why the lady is pregnant. The diaphragm holds the spermicidal jelly against the cervix so that enterprising sperm that find a way around the barrier will not survive entry into the cervix. In applying spermicide to the diaphragm, a little bit should be put on the rim because around the rim is the entryway of the sperm, and then a dollop of the jelly about the size of a fifty-cent piece is put in the bottom of the diaphragm.

One patient told me that she did not like jelly, she wanted a cream. "Most of my patients prefer the jelly," I told her.

"No, no, I want the cream." A few days later she called me. "You got the jelly?"

"Why?" I asked, knowing full well what the answer was. It was because during intercourse she resembled a hydrophobic dog as the cream came foaming out.

A diaphragm, like a dress, must be fitted to the wearer. A lady who is normally a size 18 cannot fit into a size 10 dress; it just does not work. The same holds true for a diaphragm. Some women, believing that the integrity of the vagina is reflected by the size of the diaphragm, say, "I want a smaller one. I don't want that number 80. I want a 65."

"Fine," I answer. "You want to be a mother? Does your husband want to be a father?"

The size needed is determined not by the size of the vagina but by the size of the bony pelvis. The rim has to be fitted to angle down from the pubic bone above the cervix to the sacral bone. In a large woman the bones are farther apart than in a woman who is four-foot-eleven and has small bones. If the diaphragm is too big for the woman and she can feel it, it can cause a lot of discomfort by rubbing against her sacrum or bladder. On the other hand, if the diaphragm is too small, it can easily be dislodged.

Having a diaphragm fitted in the gynecologist's office is different from putting it in place at home. In the office the environment is clinical, while the atmosphere at home is much more relaxed. That is why I tell my patients that when they get the diaphragm home, they must put it in and take it out at least ten times. "Put it in, take it out, over and over," I suggest. "You're not ready for action until you become adept at using this device. If you don't practice, you won't use the diaphragm effectively and you'll be turned off by it."

What happens at home is that the vaginal muscles relax, and sometimes the diaphragm that fit well in the office becomes uncomfortable at home, in which case the patient has to return for a refitting. I generally do a fairly tight fit in the office because I know the patient is going to be more relaxed at home, and I choose carefully between the two types of diaphragm, a flat spring and an arcing spring. For the woman who has a retroverted, that is, tilted, uterus, the flat spring is much better. An arcing spring can be uncomfortable. The latter has a firm rim that, when the rubber is pressed together, folds like a U. In contrast, the rim of the flat spring is softer, and when the edges are pressed together, they are in a straight line rather than an arc. The arcing type is the common variety; like the Graves speculum, it may be the only type an office has. But if the diaphragm feels uncomfortable or hurts, rather than give up on the idea, you should try again with a gynecologist who can supply a flat spring one.

I am not sure I should tell this story, but it does vividly prove my point about practicing ahead of time. A young engaged woman whom I fitted with a diaphragm did not get around to practicing inserting it because she was so busy with all the wedding arrangements. She packed the diaphragm in her suitcase with her going-away clothes and flew to Hawaii. When she and her new husband settled down in their hotel room, she excused herself and went into the bathroom to put the diaphragm in. Her groom lay on the bed waiting for his moment of bliss, and time passed. After half an hour he knocked on the door. "Honey, are you okay in there?"

"Yes, I'm okay."

Twenty minutes later: "Honey . . ."

"I'm not ready yet!"

"Okay, honey, I'm sorry."

The story as she told it to me: "Dr. Thornton, the thing was flying all over the bathroom. I put the jelly in and the diaphragm flipped out of my hand and landed in back of the toilet. Then it flew into the shower. There I am with one foot up on the toilet, and this thing is as slippery as an eel. It is bouncing off the bathroom mirror, off the ceiling, into the sink—everywhere but in me. It took forty-five minutes before I got it in and cleaned the jelly off the walls. So, okay, I'm finally all set and I open the bathroom door and there my new husband is—asleep! Totally asleep!"

Now you know why I tell my patients they must put a new diaphragm in and take it out ten times before they really use it. You should not go into a new adventure, into a very important time in your life, without having practiced, because that is when you get pregnant. You say, "Oh, the hell with it, I'll just put the spermicidal jelly in, that's good enough." But with a 30 percent failure rate for the jelly, it may very well not be good enough.

In general, a diaphragm can be put in place at any time. I tell my patients that when they are going out in the evening, they should put it in when they put their makeup on, that the spermicidal jelly will still be effective hours later. If there is any doubt of that, more spermicidal jelly can be added just before intercourse, which is more easily done and less interruptive than the whole diaphragm bit.

After intercourse the diaphragm must be left in place for at least eight hours, which means that if you put it in in the evening, it should be left in place until the next morning. If you have intercourse again before eight hours have gone by, do not take out the diaphragm; just add another squeeze of spermicidal jelly. The same holds true for multiple intimacies. Leave the diaphragm in place against the cervix but add jelly. Because the diaphragm is made of rubber rather than of a spongy or absorbent material that can harbor bacteria, toxic shock syndrome rarely occurs and is not a concern unless the patient has a history of toxic shock syndrome, in which case use of a diaphragm is not recommended.

When you are using a diaphragm as your contraceptive method, as time goes by you must check it for holes. Put some water in the diaphragm to see if any water droplets appear on the underside. Hold it up to the light and look for microscopic holes; sperm are tiny and they love holes. As for storing the diaphragm, the old way was to sprinkle it with talcum powder. Forget the old way. The remnants of talc clinging to the diaphragm have been associated with ovarian cancer. Instead, dust the diaphragm with cornstarch before putting it away, then rinse the starch off before inserting it.

When purchasing a diaphragm, I strongly recommend getting two—one for home, one for away. If you are a lady who travels, store one in your suitcase along with your toothbrush and pajamas; that way you will not forget it in the last-minute rush of packing. If you are working and often spend evenings in the city, keep one in the office. Spermicidal jelly is always easy to pick up in a pharmacy, but a fitted diaphragm is not.

A diaphragm may last one year or ten years, depending on how sexually active you are and how aggressive your partner is. If the diaphragm becomes discolored, if it looks ragged or old or loses its elasticity, throw it away and get another. You need not go back to your gynecologist; the pharmacy can refill your original prescription. The only time you need to be refitted is if you gain or lose more than 20 pounds or after you have had a baby.

THE CERVICAL CAP

Cervical caps are in wider use in Europe than in this country. Resembling a small version of a diaphragm, the cap fits over the cervix alone rather than covering the whole area as a diaphragm does. Unlike the diaphragm, it can be left in place for as long as 24 hours. The cervical cap is available in four different sizes and must be fitted by a professional.

Cervical caps have been suspected of being associated with abnormal cellular changes in the cervix leading to precancerous lesions. While this association has not been totally discounted, the FDA has approved their use provided that the user has a Pap smear done by her gynecologist every three months. This necessity for frequent office visits, and the fact that the cap must be properly fitted and gynecologists in this country have not had much experience with the fitting, has rather discouraged widespread use of the cap.

Another downside of both the diaphragm and cervical cap is that they can be the cause of urinary tract infections; the firm rim may irritate the delicate tissue surrounding the bladder.

THE MALE CONDOM

The condom is a thin sheath of rubber worn by the male partner over the shaft and corona (head) of the penis so that ejaculate remains contained rather than spurting into the vagina. Although the male usually does not use a spermicide with a condom, it is all to the good if the female partner does, since it increases the protection. Spermicidal condoms containing an inner and outer coating of the spermicide non-oxynol-9 are available.

As well as being marketed in a gel and a cream form, spermicides are available over the counter in tablet form. Intended for use by women, the tablets or caplets are like little suppositories for the vagina. I first learned that they can cause hypersensitivity reactions from a patient who said, "It was like my vagina was an oven. I was burning inside. I took the tablet out but I was still so hot I didn't know what to do with myself." I have since heard similar stories from other patients, so that is something to be aware of.

The important thing to remember with a condom is that the penis must still be erect when it exits the vagina. If it becomes flaccid, the penis slides out and the condom stays inside the vaginal vault. Gravity eventually causes it to fall out, but in the meantime sperm may have spilled in the vagina, necessitating emergency contraception measures.

The Female Condom. A female condom that is made out of latex and looks like the wind sock at an airport has been developed. It is a pouch that unrolls into the vagina with the penetration of the penis. Because it is awkward and as noisy as a rattling paper bag, and its effectiveness is no greater than other forms of contraception because the penis may go to the side of it, it has not been widely accepted.

THE IUD

The history of intrauterine contraceptive devices, surprisingly enough, starts with camels. Nomads in the desert traveled great distances by caravan and the caravan could not stop while a pregnant camel gave birth, so two metal balls were inserted into the womb of the female camels, which allowed them to do the wild thing whenever they had the urge but obviated the arrival of baby camels. That was the beginning of the concept of insertion of a foreign object into the uterus to prevent conception.

A page of illustrations of intrauterine devices looks like something out of a medieval manuscript. The Dalkon shield, for instance, had spines coming out of it and resembled a horseshoe crab. Some devices were rings, others bows, still others springs in every conceivable shape. Since they were not something anyone would ever see and doctors were recommending them, women accepted them. Indeed, IUDs enjoyed great popularity in the early 1970s because the device remained in place, your mother did not know of its existence, you did not have to remember to take the Pill, and you could not forget and leave it at home like a diaphragm.

Then drawbacks began to become apparent. The first IUDs had no way of being removed except by a uterine hook or a D and C. Left in place for years, the rigid object sometimes migrated, working its way through the side wall of the uterus and out into the abdomen where, if the bowel was entrapped by the ring, intestinal obstruction or perforation resulted. After this unfortunate side-effect was observed, it was decided not to make the devices rigid, not to make them in a closed shape like a circle or bow that could entrap or perforate the intestine, and to attach a string to them. That is when the Dalkon shield came along, sporting a multifilament string and little spikes or spines on its body. The string ran through the cervix and out into the vagina so that the device could be pulled out. But then it was discovered that the string acted as a superhighway for bacteria to travel from the vagina up into the uterus, and the spines made a perfect setup for infection. In 1974, 11 deaths and 209 infected abortions were attributed to use of the Dalkon shield, and the manufacturer was hit with a huge complement of product liability suits, which led to the withdrawal of the device from the market.

Subsequent generations of the IUD had monofilament strings to eliminate the easy course of bacteria into the uterus and an open design like an S-curve in a road. The Lippes loop was the best known of these, and it seemed to work well—in fact, a number of women still have a Lippes loop in place—but its use has been discontinued. Like IUDs in general, it increased the risk of ectopic pregnancy and pelvic inflammatory infection. And it was not infallible as far as contraception was concerned. I myself have delivered three babies in women with the Lippes loop in place. One loop was in the mother's abdomen, one was in the uterus as the afterbirth came out, and one was clutched in the baby's hand when it was born.

Harold Tatum of the Population Council at The Rockefeller University developed a copper device in the shape of a T, with the crosspiece fitting into the horns of the uterus. Copper makes it more effective than the polyethylene IUD, but it has to be removed after a certain period of time. All types of IUD have a 15 percent chance of causing bleeding, which then poses the question of whether the bleeding is due to the device or to a malignancy in the uterus. It is recommended that the device not be used in women over 40.

I could go on about the subsequent generations of IUDs and their problems and the fact that the cost rose to six hundred dollars or so to have one inserted, plus the cost of having it removed if the string broke and the cost of major surgery if the device worked its way into the abdomen, versus the cost of a diaphragm or the Pill—but enough has been said to make it clear why IUDs have fallen into disfavor.

If you are a woman who has a Lippes loop or any other discontinued IUD in place and you are beyond childbearing age, I would suggest you have the device removed because of its tendency to increase the chances of infection and because it can cause uterine perforation by burrowing its way through the wall of the uterus into the abdominal cavity. If the string has broken on your IUD, an ultrasound examination is needed to identify its location. Curettage can remove it from the uterus, but if the IUD has migrated and is extrauterine, that calls for major surgery.

Today in the United States, only two IUDs are approved by the FDA: TCu 380A and Progestasert. TCu 380A is a T-shaped device made of polyurethane wound with copper wire; it is approved for eight years of continuous use. Progestasert is also T-shaped, but it contains progesterone in oil which is slowly released into the system over a period of time and adds to the effectiveness of the device. It is approved for only one year of continuous contraception. IUDs are usually inserted at the time of the menses to minimize the discomfort of insertion and to avoid insertion in the midst of an early pregnancy. They are effective immediately.

STERILIZATION

As noted, the most common form of contraception among couples is sterilization of either the man or the woman. Because in the final analysis whoever carries the child is the one who is going to be the one most concerned about birth control, it is more usually the wife than the husband who elects sterilization. I have known women to have seven or eight cesarean sections and still the husband will not have a vasectomy—because "I don't want to be less of a man." This is an emotional rather than a rational response; sterilization in the male does not affect potency, and the procedure is far simpler and less risky for the male than for the female.

A vasectomy can be done in the doctor's office under local anesthesia. It is a very simple urological procedure that takes only 45 minutes. In contrast, a bilateral tubal ligation and resection in a woman is an in-hospital procedure carried out under general or epidural anesthesia. That, at least, is the humane way; some women allow themselves to be convinced that it can be done under local anesthesia, but it has to be a sadist who puts a woman through that.

When the procedure is done in the hospital operating room, the

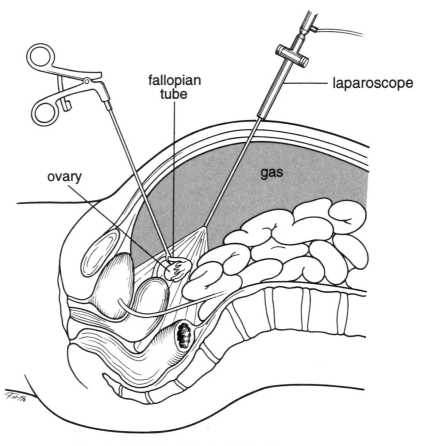

ovary　　　fallopian　　laparoscope
　　　　　　tube

gas

Female Tubal Sterilization Using Laparoscope

surgeon first inflates the abdomen with carbon dioxide and then goes in with a laparoscope to visualize the fallopian tubes and occlude them by cautery (high heat) or tie them off. If all goes well, it is same-day surgery. As in any invasive procedure, there are risks involved—in this case, laceration of the bowel, bleeding, and infection.

The procedure can be done immediately postpartum. After the baby is delivered, the uterus usually remains high enough in the abdomen for the next 24 hours for a small incision to be made underneath the navel and for the tubes to be grasped, surgically tied, and cut. If the procedure is not done within a day, or at most two, however, there is a risk of postpartum infection, so the surgery must be postponed until at least six weeks after delivery; by that time the uterus has returned to its normal small size and laparoscopy is needed.

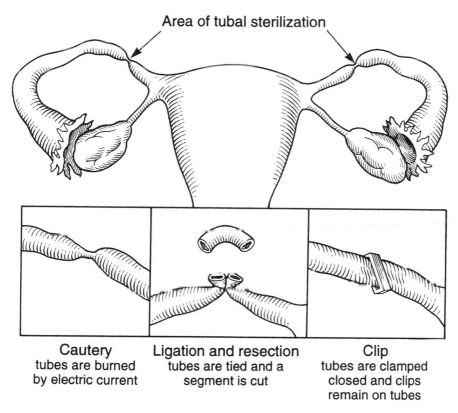

Area of tubal sterilization

| Cautery
tubes are burned
by electric current | Ligation and resection
tubes are tied and a
segment is cut | Clip
tubes are clamped
closed and clips
remain on tubes |

Types of Tubal Sterilization

The failure rate for both male and female sterilization is the same failure rate meaning the occurrence of an unintended pregnancy. Even with tied tubes or vasectomy, there is a three to four per thousand chance of pregnancy. Put another way, protection is 99.96 percent certain but not 100 percent. The failure comes if, in the case of a vasectomy, the sperm count is still there, or if, in the case of a tubal ligation, a tiny fistula, or opening, develops above the point where the tube has been cut and tied, allowing the sperm to meet the egg. Sperm and egg are a powerful pair; they find each other like heat-seeking missiles despite the best efforts of human beings to keep them apart.

When I began practicing at The New York Hospital in the 1980s, one of my patients was a woman who had seven children. Three of the births were by cesarean section, all of them were complicated and difficult, and the mother almost lost her life with the seventh baby. She wanted to have her tubes tied but she could not have it done unless her husband signed a paper giving his consent. I questioned why she needed his consent when he did not need hers to have a vasectomy. The answer was "Because that's the way it's always been done here at New York Hospital."

"Not fair," said I. "Not right." It turned out that no one had ever questioned the rule before, and when I did, it was rescinded. That is one of the benefits of having more and more women entering the field of medicine: Accepted practices that no one gave any thought to before are being questioned—and often discarded as unfair or outmoded.

RHYTHM METHOD

The rhythm or natural family planning method is based on predicting the fertile period of a woman's cycle and on her abstention from sex during that time frame. To determine when ovulation occurs involves daily charting by the woman of her basal body temperature, which rises by half a degree after ovulation. An alternate or supplemental method is the cervical mucus, or Billings, method in which the woman collects mucus from her vagina and examines its characteristics to see if it is clear and stretchy or slippery; if so, it indicates that she is about to ovulate.

Once a patient has learned when to expect the time of ovulation, she can calculate her fertile period, which is seven days before ovulation and four days after, and abstain from intercourse during this time. Unfortunately, not every woman has an undeviating monthly cycle in which her period comes exactly every 28 or every 30 days, and even if she does, the sperm can hang around for five to seven days waiting for ovulation to occur.

With a failure rate approaching 25 percent, the rhythm method is not a particularly effective form of contraception, but it is an approach utilized by women who, for religious or other reasons, do not wish to employ alternate means. The method has no side-effects or contraindications, except perhaps for two weeks of frustration every month.

EMERGENCY CONTRACEPTION

A hormone regimen using the birth control pill can be effective in preventing pregnancy if taken within 72 hours of *one* episode of unprotected intercourse (the Yuzpe method). The regimen most frequently prescribed is a double dose of a specific birth control pill, followed by another double dose 12 hours later. The specific birth control pill is prescribed by your gynecologist or women's clinic. This emergency contraception is thought to prevent pregnancy by suppressing ovulation or altering the transport of the egg through the fallopian tube. The failure rate is only one to two percent. The Reproductive Health Technologies Project's hotline to inform women of emergency contraception is 1-800-584-9911.

There are downsides to all the contraceptives. I have seen mini-strokes in women taking the Pill, ectopic pregnancies and pelvic inflammatory disease in women using IUDs, and keloidal scars on the arms of ladies with implants. Occasionally, I want to cry out: "Why do women have to accept all the risk? When is there going to be a male contraceptive?" But I know the answer. Never. Men do not have the babies. Nobody is interested in developing a male contraceptive, and if a drug company did, men would not be inclined to use it because it is not men who get pregnant. So, women have to choose among the methods available and hope that the perfect one, unfailing and without side-effects, will someday be found.

POINTS TO REMEMBER

- Mother Nature does not intend to have the human race die out. Thus, there is no contraceptive method that is guaranteed never to fail.
- Don't trust to luck. Eighty-five percent of women who do become pregnant.
- If you use a diaphragm, do not forget the spermicidal jelly. And practice inserting it before you use it in earnest.
- Put your diaphragm in when you put your makeup on, and leave the diaphragm in place for eight hours after intercourse.
- When a condom is the contraceptive device being used, the male must exit while the penis is still erect.
- Women who have an intrauterine device in place should have it removed when they are beyond childbearing age.
- The Pill is still the least traumatic, most effective, reversible contraceptive method. It should be taken at the same time every day. No woman should smoke while on the Pill.

II

PREGNANCY

❧

5

I'M PREGNANT

❧

HOME PREGNANCY TEST • DATING A PREGNANCY • TALKING ABOUT PREGNANCY • EATING FOR TWO • DIET IN PREGNANCY • WATER • MILK • FRUIT • FISH • MEAT • VEGETABLES • EGGS AND CHEESE • A FOOD DIARY • ALCOHOL • SMOKING • COFFEE • EXERCISE DURING PREGNANCY • WORKING DURING PREGNANCY • OVER-THE-COUNTER MEDICATIONS • COLDS • HEADACHES • VITAMINS • X-RAYS AND MICROWAVES • ENVIRONMEN- TAL HAZARDS • MORNING SICKNESS • VAGINAL BLEED-ING • IMPLANTATION BLEEDING • ECTOPIC PREGNANCY • MISCARRIAGE • BLEEDING LATE IN PREGNANCY • BED REST • MULTIPLE GESTATIONS • SELECTIVE REDUCTION •

The process in pregnancy is this: The egg erupts from the ovary, and the fimbria, which are the fringelike ends of a fallopian tube, sweep over the ovary and vacuum it up. The egg starts down the tube, and the sperm comes up from the vagina into the uterus to meet the egg in the last third of the fallopian tube and fertilize it. The fertilized conceptus then rolls down the tube into the uterus. It has immedi-ately started to divide into two cells, and the two cells become four cells. Originally it is called a morula, then it becomes a blastocyte, and that blastocyte begins to burrow into the endometrial lining. From this beginning, the miracle is that nine months later out comes a fat little baby, breathing and kicking and yelling.

HOME PREGNANCY TEST

A home pregnancy test affords privacy, and that is why it is so popular. You don't have to go to the doctor, you don't have to wait to get an appointment, you don't have to let anyone know that you suspect you might be pregnant. You make a trip to the pharmacy, pick up the test, take it back home, and pee. The test is either positive or negative; you are pregnant or you are not.

The test is highly sensitive to the presence of human chorionic gonadotropin (hCG), the pregnancy hormone. What it does not reveal, however, is where the pregnancy is. It can be in a fallopian tube, but you, like most women, assume it is in its proper place in the uterus and you figure you will finish the project you are working on or you will take the vacation that has been planned and go to the doctor later. The next thing you know you have fainted and have a belly full of blood from a ruptured ectopic pregnancy.

No test in and of itself diagnoses an ectopic pregnancy, but what the doctor does is a serum blood test to determine the level of hCG and compare that with a subsequent blood test in two or three days. The level of hCG should double every forty-eight hours. If, for instance, it starts out at 10,000, in two days it should be at 20,000. If it is not—if it is at 11,000 instead—the possibility of an ectopic pregnancy is there and a very close watch is kept on the patient.

Another warning sign is spotting. Vaginal spotting is similar to the final days of a period when the blood flow is light and intermittent. The spotting can be implantation bleeding (described later), or the patient may assume it is mittelschmerz, but since it is also one of the early signs of ectopic pregnancy, it should bring the patient to the doctor. We know what the level of hCG should be at every gestational age, and if a blood test shows it to be lower than expected, the question is whether it is an ectopic pregnancy or a pregnancy on its way out—that is, a spontaneous abortion or miscarriage. If at six weeks hCG is at three times the level expected, the possibility of a molar pregnancy, a gestational mole, is present. Rare in the United States but common in the Philippines, a mole is a buildup of trophoblastic tissue, something that occurs when the trophoblasts, which are the villi that are supposed to anchor a fetus, go haywire and start multiplying in the absence of a pregnancy. The patient requires a D and C so that this trophoblastic disease does not metastasize to other parts of the body. It can become malignant and go to the patient's lungs and brain, and it is a terrible thing. Suffice it to say, if you have a positive pregnancy test, the next step, not to be delayed, is to see an obstetrician who will differentiate between a molar pregnancy, an impending spontaneous miscarriage, an ectopic pregnancy, and the one we all know, an intrauterine pregnancy.

Once upon a time I was opposed to home pregnancy tests because of these other possibilities, but I have come to understand a woman's urgent need to know, either because she is so eager to become pregnant or because she is fearful that she may be pregnant. I do want to convey, however, how important it is to see a doctor promptly. This is true even if the pregnancy test is negative because you should seek medical advice about why your period is late. It still can be an ectopic pregnancy that is not producing high enough numbers to make the test positive. The bottom line is: What are you waiting around for? Your periods have been regular, now you have missed a period or it has been irrregular, and you need to be evaluated in a systematic way.

I have been accused of coming on too strongly about this, but only by people who have not seen dead women, women who should be alive but are not because they got the wrong advice or waited too long.

DATING A PREGNANCY

In modern obstetrics, we no longer date a pregnancy in months; it is not accurate enough. Instead we date it in weeks. Forty weeks is equal to ten lunar months, which is equal to nine calendar months. A lunar month has 28 days or four weeks in it, while a calendar month has 30 or 31 days. Therefore, the nine months of pregnancy are really 40 weeks. A full-term baby is mature between 38 and 42 weeks of gestation.

The clock starts ticking from the time of the first day of your last menstrual period, not when you conceived. The pregnancy is then divided into trimesters. The first trimester runs from the first day of your last menstrual period to 12 weeks. The second trimester is 12 weeks to 28 weeks, and the third trimester is 28 weeks until the time the baby is born at 38 to 42 weeks.

TALKING ABOUT PREGNANCY

Society puts a great deal of pressure on women to have babies, to bring on the next generation, and women themselves, whether con-

sciously or not, take pride in proving themselves fertile. It is not surprising, then, that the minute there is a positive pregnancy test, the
whole town is likely to hear about it. The woman tells everyone,
"I'm pregnant! I'm pregnant!" When she has a miscarriage, however,
few people hear about it, which is why there is a general mispercep-
tion about the frequency of miscarriages. The public tends to believe
they are rare, while in fact 25 to 30 percent of pregnancies do not
make it past the twelfth week.

If at eight weeks you are telling people, "I'm pregnant," you have
a one-in-three or -four chance at 12 weeks of having to tell them, "I
miscarried," and having to deal with the questions. It is bad enough
to be asking yourself: "What did I do? What did the doctor do?
What did my husband do? What did that taxicab driver do?" without
having to field other people's queries. I feel that it is not good, not
healthy, to put yourself through that. I tell my patients not to tell
anyone they are pregnant until they are 26 weeks along. If anything
happens at that time we can save the baby, but before 26 weeks, if
nature intervenes with bleeding or ruptured membranes or preterm
labor, the baby is lost and you have to un-tell everyone that you told
about your pregnancy. If some of your friends have gone off in the
meantime to Boston or the Caribbean or the West Coast, every time
one returns, it has all to be gone through again: "How is the baby?"
"Well, we lost it." The emotional toll is high every time another
person must be told. It is like having a bruise that does not heal
because you keep getting hit in the same place over and over.

If you are strong enough and your husband is strong enough, the
best thing is to say to yourselves: We conceived this baby, we are
happy about it, why does everyone else need to know about it? If you
tell one person, you might as well tell the whole world because that
one person is going to tell a couple of others in confidence, and they
will tell a couple of others, and so on. Yes, it is tempting for a man to
brag, "I'm going to be a father," and it is tempting for a woman
to brag, "I'm going to be a mother." But the bragging can come back
to haunt you both if the pregnancy does not end with a full-term,
healthy baby.

In short, in my opinion, whoever was not present when the baby
was conceived should not be told about your pregnancy until you are
26 weeks along. Does this include your mother and your sister? If
you are my patient, I hope it does because I had rather you listened

to my advice than theirs. Case in point: I will say you shouldn't take aspirin, and your mother will say, "Why not? I took aspirin when I was carrying you." I will say you must not smoke, and your mother will say, "I smoked when I was pregnant. That's why I had small babies and didn't need a cesarean."

I recently had a patient who had a very complicated pregnancy because she is a diabetic and on insulin. She needed to be delivered, but because insulin-dependent diabetes is known to delay fetal lung maturity, we first needed to do an amniocentesis to determine whether the baby's lungs had developed to the point where it could survive. We scheduled the patient for this, but then she called in tears. "My mother said not to have the amnio. It might kill the baby. She knows three women who had amnio late and the baby died the next day." I reassured her as best I could, and we went ahead with the amniocentesis because it was the appropriate thing to do, but that mother had reduced her daughter to a state of high anxiety and made her go through an agony of worry that was not necessary.

Offhand comments from people who consider themselves authorities on pregnancy because they have had a couple of children are troublesome because the practice of obstetrics has progressed so rapidly and become so much more sophisticated in just a short period of time that what was happening 20 or 30 years ago is simply not applicable now. Listening to the pronouncements can mislead the patient and cause her conflict and upset.

Having been in practice for some years, I see the same patients over time. With their first pregnancy, they pay no attention to my advice to keep mum until it is showing, but with a second pregnancy, they tend to be like a patient of mine. "You know what I'm going to tell you," I said when her pregnancy was confirmed.

"You don't have to. I got so sick of hearing from every side during my first pregnancy that I'm not telling anyone about this one. I could hardly bring myself to tell my husband, and I swore him to secrecy."

Nobody knew she was pregnant, and she went along without any aggravation until 26 weeks, when people started saying, "Are you gaining weight or something?" and she answered, "Oh, yeah, I'm pregnant. Didn't you know?" That released the flood of unsolicited advice, but now she was primed to ignore it.

It is wondrously strange but people give advice like: A little bleeding? Don't worry. A few pains? Don't go to the hospital until you really feel . . . The waters broke? Get into the bathtub and relax. Have some blackberry brandy until you get a little groggy. Meanwhile, the umbilical cord has prolapsed and is in the bathtub and the baby is in trouble. People should hold their tongues. If they are not obstetricians, if they have not seen thousands of women, if they are ignorant of the dark side of obstetrics, they should say no more than, "You're pregnant? Wonderful! Let's have a cup of tea to celebrate."

EATING FOR TWO

I wish I knew where that phrase came from. I suppose it has been around since the beginning of time, but it is the bane of the obstetrical world. Why? Because women get too fat. "I'm pregnant and have to eat for two now. Dear, would you nip down to the convenience store and get a quart of Häagen-Dazs?" This kind of reasoning is wrong and unhealthful. Just because you are pregnant is no reason to gain quantities of weight. No one would say to a person who had just had a total hip replacement, "Okay, gain 60 pounds." On the contrary, you'd say, "You're going to put a lot of stress on that hip. Please make sure you hold your weight at a reasonable level."

Alas, we obstetricians do not often say that to our patients. We are just as culpable as the general public because we are human too. Before we arrived at medical school, we listened to our mothers and grandmothers talking and picked up their information. A scientific education got larded on top, but the old sayings lingered on underneath, and since nutrition is not the forte of medical schools, there was little there to gainsay them. That is why doctors say, "You gained five pounds? Don't worry about it." And when the patient asks, "How much should I gain?" the reply is likely to be, "You're doing okay."

The fact of the matter is that you are not eating for two, you are eating for one and a twentieth. A baby at term weighs six or seven pounds; if you are a 140-pound woman, that seven-pound baby is one-twentieth the size of you, so there is no reason in the world to eat for two you's.

You should gain only two pounds in the first trimester. At 12 weeks, the baby weighs 14 grams. An ounce is 30 grams, so 14 is not even half an ounce, which means there is no excuse for a ten-pound weight gain.

After the first trimester, weight gain should be three-quarters of a pound to one pound per week for the remainder of the pregnancy, for a total weight gain during pregnancy of 21 to 26 pounds.

Why that much even? Because there is a baby in there, which makes for seven pounds. Then there is the weight of the placenta (1¹/₂ lbs), the amniotic fluid (2 lbs), and the increased size and weight of the uterus (2¹/₂ lbs). The breasts, affected by hormones, become about one pound heavier. The blood volume is increased in pregnancy (3¹/₂ lbs), as is the deposition of fat, which should be held to 6 or 7 pounds. A lot of structural changes do occur in pregnancy. But they do not add up to 65 pounds' worth.

The single most important source of complications in pregnancy, in my opinion, is excessive weight gain. The complications range from gestational diabetes to toxemia or preeclampsia, to large babies requiring delivery by cesarean section or other operative types of delivery, i.e., forceps and vacuum extraction, and to postpartum depression after the baby is born. Recent studies published in the *Journal of the American Medical Association* have even linked obesity in pregnancy with an increase in the incidence of neural tube defects (spina bifida). Although, as I say, the normal baby at term is between six and seven pounds, that size is almost a peanut these days because women are going hog-wild and gaining 50, 60, 70, or 80 pounds. Perhaps this is in reaction to the 1950s when women were told to gain no more than 10 pounds and babies were coming out at five pounds. Ten pounds was too restrictive, just as 50 pounds is too liberal. The middle course, which is what we obstetricians are recommending now, is 26 pounds. Thirty is still all right, but if you tell a woman 30 she will go to 40.

Most people are not obstetricians and they want to see pregnant women fat. The pregnant woman walks into an elevator or a store or a meeting and everyone says, "When are you due?" Even though she knows that if she weren't pregnant, they wouldn't ask her for the time of day, she wants to be polite and so she answers, "Next month."

"You're due next month? You don't look that big. Are you okay?"

That's when the obstetrician gets the call. The patient has gained 22 pounds and she is doing great. She has a month to go, and at the rate of a pound a week, she will be at 26 pounds at delivery, just where she should be. But in the interval between being told she looks small and calling her obstetrician, she has downed two eclairs and a milkshake because now she is listening to the general public. With luck, the obstetrician will convince her that the general public is not a good judge of these matters.

The weight gain should be just in the abdomen, not under the arms, not on the thighs, not under the jowls. There has been a lot of talk about "unnecessary cesarean sections," but if you have a nine-pound baby, a cesarean section may be needed to deliver it. And who made that nine-pound kid? The mother whose eating habits went out of control: "I only gained 72 pounds. I figure I can lose it later."

Losing those pounds later may prove to be impossible. Before the baby arrived, you had time and energy to go to the gym, but now you have a baby and who is going to take care of it while you are at the spa? Your maternal instincts kick in and you want to be there with your child, especially if you are breast-feeding. Your whole life changes, and your intention to get back to your prepregnancy weight goes by the board.

Weight Watchers has a pregnancy and nursing weight control plan that can go a long way in ensuring that you and your baby are healthy. Say a woman starts her pregnancy at 270 pounds—some women do, believe me. They come to the office with an agenda already in mind. "Now, you know, Dr. Thornton, I'm supposed to gain 25 pounds. That's what my previous doctor told me."

"Not when you come in here six weeks pregnant at 270 pounds. You're going to go on this program—not a diet, *a program.* You're going to write down everything you eat for the remainder of this pregnancy, and what you eat is going to be this number of servings of fruit, this number of servings of vegetables, et cetera. If you find that you are losing weight but I find that you are healthy, I don't care about the weight loss. You're gaining nutrients, the baby is gaining nutrients, and you are losing excess fat."

One lady, who came in at 302 pounds, began losing weight on the Weight Watchers program. She said, "I'm not listening to the people who tell me I should be putting on weight," and I told her, "Fine, you just listen to me." By the time I delivered her daughter, the woman was down to 280, and after she delivered, she went on to lose another 40 pounds. She and her daughter were both the healthier for it.

Modern medicine no longer uses height, weight, and frame in arriving at what is considered to be overweight and what is not. Nutritionists and bariatricians (specialists in weight) now use the body mass index (BMI) as the standard. The BMI divides your weight in kilograms by your height in meters squared. The calculations have been done for you in Table 2. According to the BMI, you are underweight at 19.8, normal if the BMI is between 19.8 and 26, plump if it is between 26 and 29, and obese if it is more than 29.

TABLE 2

Body Mass Index

Height	Underweight if BMI <20 wt. less than	Normal BMI 20–26 between	Overweight BMI 26–29 between	Obese BMI >29 wt. greater than
4'8"	89	89–112	112–125	125
4'9"	92	92–117	117–130	130
4'10"	95	95–124	124–138	138
4'11"	99	99–128	128–143	143
5'0"	102	102–133	133–148	148
5'1"	106	106–137	137–153	153
5'2"	109	109–142	142–158	158
5'3"	113	113–146	146–163	163
5'4"	116	116–151	151–169	169
5'5"	120	120–156	156–174	174
5'6"	124	124–161	161–179	179
5'7"	127	127–166	166–185	185
5'8"	131	131–171	171–190	190
5'9"	135	135–176	176–196	196
5'10"	139	139–181	181–202	202
5'11"	143	143–186	186–208	208
6'0"	147	147–192	192–214	214
6'1"	151	151–196	196–219	219
6'2"	155	155–203	203–226	226
6'3"	160	160–207	207–231	231
6'4"	164	164–214	214–238	238
6'5"	168	168–217	217–242	242

DIET IN PREGNANCY

Water. A pregnant woman needs to drink eight glasses of water a day—not tea or coffee or soda, but clear, cool water. In the summer it should be ten glasses a day because of the water lost in increased perspiration. I tell my patients to fill two quart containers with water and put them in the refrigerator. Take one to work with you and drink one in the evening at home. Then fill both of them back up so they chill overnight and are ready for the next day. That way you quantify exactly how much you are drinking. Doing so is important because not drinking enough water is thought to be a prime cause of preterm (premature) labor.

When it is time for a baby to be born, a hormone called oxytocin stimulates the uterine musculature to initiate contractions. This hormone is secreted in the paraventricular nucleus of the hypothalamus, a gland in the brain. Right next to the paraventricular nucleus is the supraoptic nucleus. The paraventricular nucleus is responsible for oxytocin and the supraoptic nucleus for an antidiuretic hormone. The antidiuretic—*anti* meaning against, *diuresis* meaning urination—hormone kicks in when you are dehydrated; it tells your body, "Hold on to the water in the body. Don't urinate it out." The supraoptic nucleus gets excited because it is secreting all that antidiuretic hormone, and next to it the paraventricular nucleus picks up the excitation and begins secreting oxytocin. All of a sudden: "I'm having contractions! I'm in labor!"

The treatment for preterm labor is to hospitalize the patient and administer a liter of fluid intravenously over a period of time, something that would not be necessary if she had drunk a quart of water that day. With hydration the contractions usually calm right down.

Milk. In addition to the two quarts of water a day, you should have one quart of skim milk. Not whole milk, skim milk, because it has no fat and, believe it or not, it contains more calcium than whole milk; I don't know why, but it does. If you are lactose-intolerant and cannot take milk, two eight-ounce servings of fat-free yogurt is a good equivalent. If you drink two quarts of water and a quart of milk a day, you won't wonder if you can get away with having a soda, a milkshake, or a glass of fruit juice. You won't have room for it.

Milk is important because there is a little person in there building bones and teeth for which calcium is needed. Furthermore, if you get adequate amounts of calcium, your own risk of developing osteoporosis in later life is lessened. Women say, "I don't like milk. I'll just take a calcium tablet," but there is more in milk than just calcium, and a tablet does not substitute for the proteins, vitamins, and minerals that are also important for the growing fetus. (See chapter 21, table 7.)

Fruit. Fruit juices are concentrated sweets. An 8-ounce glass of orange juice is about 120 calories, and who drinks only an 8-ounce glass? Without even realizing it, you'll slurp up 300 calories and then wonder why you are gaining weight. "All I'm drinking is fruit juice, and they say that's good for you." No, it's not. The whole fruit is what is good for you. Take an orange, spend the time to peel it, savor it as you eat it, benefit from the pulp and the fiber that keep you from becoming constipated, and rejoice that it is only 80 calories as opposed to 300. Do the same with an apple rather than drink apple juice or cider. Eat five whole fruits a day, and for something to drink, stick to water.

Fish. At least five of the 21 meals you eat per week should be fish because fish is low in calories and high in protein, and protein is good for the baby you are making. But stay away from the scavengers of the sea, clams and scallops and oysters; they may carry hepatitis. Shrimp and lobster are acceptable, but not the butter that goes with the lobster.

Meat. Red meat is high in cholesterol, high in fat, and low in fiber. The occasional hamburger or steak is okay, but eat them sparingly and substitute more chicken and turkey. Pork and veal are all right. It is marbled fat that is to be avoided.

Vegetables. The concern with vegetables is to eat plenty of them but not the ones with hidden sugar; peas, corn, onions, and beets should be eaten minimally. If a patient is gaining too much weight and happens to mention that she loves corn on the cob, I can guess that that is where the extra calories are coming from.

Eggs and Cheese. No more than four eggs a week. As for cheese, pregnant women tend to become little mice; they love it. But cheese has fat and a high sodium content, and again the word is to eat it sparingly. Four slices of hard cheese a week, that's about it, although there is no limit on pot cheese or cottage cheese; you can have as much of these as you wish.

A Food Diary. It is an excellent idea to write down everything you eat because if you are losing weight, your doctor can see from your diary whether your diet is nevertheless a good and proper one, and if you are gaining weight, you both can check where you are going wrong. It also reinforces your willpower. A craving to eat half a layer cake can seem irresistible until you visualize having to write it down. Actually, I tell my patients that I would rather they have the cake than say to themselves, "I can't have it. I *can't* have it" and torture themselves with craving. "You can have it," I tell them, "as long as you write it down and bring your diary every time you come to see me."

Going over the diary with the patient gives us something to talk about. After the first 13 weeks, about all the obstetrician has to do is tummy checks. The nurse weighs the patient and gets a urine sample. The obstetrician has only to measure the abdominal height and listen to the baby's heart, and the patient is out of there in five minutes. But I like to keep my patients longer, and weight and food are irresistible topics of conversation. We go over the patient's food diary and I say, "What happened here?"

"Well, you see, I went to this party . . ."

"Uh-huh . . ."

"I won't do it again, I promise."

"I hope not, because what you eat in these few months you are pregnant will have an impact on 110 years of life: forty years of your life and 70 years of the life you are making."

My patients don't always like me for my strictness about diet. A lot of them have friends who are pregnant at the same time, and they come in saying, "My friend's doctor said she doesn't have to worry about her weight."

My answer is: "Your friend and her doctor are responsible for her baby. You and I are responsible for your baby. Please listen to me. You may not like it now, but I promise you that you will later."

And later the patient comes back and says, "You know, I really hated you, you were too strict, but now I have to say thank you. Why? Because my baby is healthy, number one. Number two, I can get back into my jeans, while my friend is in a postpartum depression because she is so heavy."

Alcohol. None at all during pregnancy. Absolutely no drinking—not wine, not beer, not liquor. Women who are wine drinkers will protest that wine is good for them, that it brings down the "bad" LDL cholesterol and increases the "good" HDL cholesterol. (See chapter 20.) The answer to that is, when you are pregnant the estrogen being secreted is increasing your HDL and lowering your LDL; you are protected naturally.

What is not protected is your baby, because the fetus does not have the enzyme that breaks down alcohol. Adult livers have alcohol dehydrogenase, which detoxifies alcohol, but the fetal liver lacks it. We do not know the effect of even one glass of alcohol on a specific fetus. Maybe it will do okay, or maybe it is a fetus whose growth is going to be affected. Maybe the mother's liver will break the alcohol down entirely, or maybe enough will reach the baby to produce fetal alcohol syndrome.

Sometimes a mother does not admit to the obstetrician that she is drinking, but then when her baby is born, it has the distinct facial features of fetal alcohol syndrome: a flat, broad nose, thin lips, and an epicanthal, or mongoloid, fold of the eyes. Mental retardation can be significant because the alcohol has affected the brain. The doctor asks the mother if she has been tippling, and now she acknowledges that indeed she has.

My feeling is that if everything happens not to turn out all right with the baby, there is enough guilt already in the mix without the mother having to recognize that behavior under her control has damaged her child. How much better it is for the mother to be able to say, "I'm not taking any chances. I'm going to do it the right way. Then if something happens, it's the fault of nature—I did everything I could."

But people are stubborn, and there are always the ones who say, "I'm going to do what I want because I know my baby's going to be perfect." To them I make the only answer I can: "It's not my baby. I am going home to my own family after I deliver your baby. But if your baby comes out with mental retardation or is physically handicapped because of something you did or did not do, it is your child. And it is going to be your child for a lifetime, not just for a few weeks."

Put that way, many patients will say, "I never thought about the long haul, Dr. Thornton. All right, I won't take chances."

Smoking. Cigarette smoke contains carbon monoxide as well as tar and nicotine, and these noxious substances cause constriction of the blood vessels. With that constriction, oxygen and nutrients do not flow as freely across the placenta as they normally would, making for smaller-than-average babies. This used to be called intrauterine fetal growth retardation (IUGR), but parents focused on the word retardation, linking it with mental retardation, so it is now called intrauterine fetal growth restriction. This restriction does not apply just to the newborn. When he or she starts school, the child is usually shorter than his classmates, and this discrepancy most likely will continue throughout life.

Also throughout their lives, the children of mothers who smoke have an increased incidence of asthma and respiratory problems. This is true even if the mother is not a smoker herself but lives in a smoking environment. In taking a history, I ask not just whether the patient smokes but whether her husband does, whether her friends do, and whether she is in a smoking environment at work. If the answer to any of these questions is yes, she has to school herself to be firm and say: "Honey, if you want to smoke, please do it outside" or "I can't come over to your house because it's a smoking house" or "I can't work in this situation."

The same holds true for marijuana, not because it is rumored to cause chromosomal breaks but because of the smoke itself and its effect on the vessels of the placenta.

Coffee. A cup of coffee a day is acceptable. In fact, I urge it on patients who have trouble moving their bowels and feel they need that cup of coffee to get them going. But not a mug, a cup. Caffeine is okay in moderation, as is everything else except alcohol and cigarettes. Even ice cream is fine as long as you have a serving, not a vat.

Among the more esoteric things you should not have are black licorice, which reportedly causes hypertension, and sassafras tea, which is said to cause uterine contractions.

EXERCISE DURING PREGNANCY

Walking is the perfect exercise. But that is walking half an hour a day in the open air, not walking back and forth to the copy machine in an office. If the weather is inclement, a stationary bicycle is an excellent substitute. Swimming, too, is good if there is a pool available.

Driving is acceptable if you wear a seat belt and if you can get your abdomen behind the wheel, but you should get out of the car and walk around every hour; otherwise, the blood flow stagnates because of the angle of the hip joint and the cramping of the uterus in the confined space. The same considerations apply when flying in a plane. Get up frequently and walk in the aisles on flights of two or three hours. As for longer flights, a pregnant woman should not be on them.

WORKING DURING PREGNANCY

How are so many women able to keep on working when they are pregnant? They are troopers. They grit their teeth and somehow keep going. But I am not sure we should applaud them because the worst thing a woman can do when she is pregnant is not to get sufficient rest. I tell my patients this: You are doing as big a job as your husband and his coworkers combined. It is as though you are building a whole city within your body. From something that starts out the size of the head of a pin, you are building a seven-pound kid, and that takes a lot of labor and effort. Nobody can see it, but your body is working hard and it gets exhausted, twice as exhausted if you overextend yourself physically, if you say, "I can do it all—work, run a house, have a baby. After all, my great-grandmother was out in the fields behind the oxen."

Do you know how many babies were lost in your great grandmother's day? A lot. People then had twelve and thirteen children: "Well, we lost this one. We'll start again next month." But that is no longer our attitude. Now every baby is a premium kid. Women who are on their feet all day—nurses, cashiers, salespeople—are at much higher risk of going into premature labor than women who can lie down for some part of the day.

If your lifestyle is such that it will jeopardize your having a full-term baby, then it is time to rethink what you are doing. A case in point: A 44-year-old actress on a television series was pregnant with twins and said she intended to keep on working right up to the time she was showing. When I heard that, I remarked to my husband, "Preterm birth, what do you want to bet?" The next night I was in the checkout line at the supermarket and there was the headline: "Dr. Quinn, Medicine Woman, collapses on the set." Sure enough, she went on to deliver prematurely.

This is not to put a guilt trip on women who genuinely cannot change their work or give it up. But they really need to think seriously about what is going on. There are physiological changes in your body. These changes don't care about your financial status. They just know that if you are not getting enough oxygen, not getting enough water, not getting enough rest, they may well push this baby out prematurely.

In 1980 we obstetricians said we had to find a way to stop premature labor because so many women were having 28-week, 7-month babies and it was costing billions of dollars to pull these infants through. To this end, tocolytic medications—*tocos* meaning contractions, *lytic* meaning to stop—were developed. That was in 1980. Now it is 1996 and we still have the same level of preterm births as in 1980. Why? I believe it is because so many women are overdoing it in the workplace.

To some extent, the risk involved in work depends on what type of work you do. However, having a desk job is not the answer unless you remember not to sit still for more than an hour at a time. You have to get up, walk around, get a glass of water, go to the ladies' room. If you're a taxi driver, you have to get out of the car and walk around. If you work in an airline terminal and you're lifting bags, you must change jobs. If you are an executive, you should not be jetting from coast to coast.

A woman threatened with premature labor needs to be on bed rest. She needs to have her feet up. She needs to lie on her side. And she needs to drink at least 8 to 10 glasses of water a day to keep well hydrated. Instead, she says, "Give me the pill that's for preterm labor. I have to be back at work on Monday." When I ask why, she answers, "Because I only have disability insurance for two weeks."

I am not unsympathetic but I have to say, "Your body is obviously telling you that you must relax, and if you don't listen to it, all the medication in the world is not going to help."

Not only is it not going to help but tocolytic medications have a downside. The woman's pulse rate goes up to 120 beats a minute and her heart begins pumping hard because drugs such as ritodrine are analogues of adrenaline. What does adrenaline have to do with stopping contractions? The hypothesis is that, in times long past, labor progressed unless the woman was threatened by sudden danger and had to take flight. Then the adrenaline pumped out in the fight-or-flight reaction slowed down labor until the danger was past and she was once again in a safe place to give birth.

When steady, painful contractions occur before 37 weeks and are strong enough to dilate the cervix to 2 centimeters, the diagnosis of preterm labor is made. Because ritodrine has been associated with an increased rate of complications in the mother, other medications are often tried first, such as magnesium sulfate, terbutaline (an asthma medication), or Procardia (a calcium-channel blocker). After 33 completed weeks of pregnancy, delivery of the baby is usually preferable because these tocolytic medications can have serious side-effects for the mother, from heart irregularities to fluid in the lung. At 33 weeks, the baby weighs at least four pounds and should suffer from no major problems.

I am an obstetrician so I am a fetal advocate, and I strongly believe that we have to get our priorities straight. To give the baby the best possible chance of going to full term, there have to be changes in a working woman's life. They are not easy changes. They are financial and they are emotional. But when a woman is pregnant, the baby is doing the talking and she would do well to listen. There are far too many preterm births, with their heightened risk to the health and well-being of both mother and child and the economic cost to society of the tremendous medical effort expended in attempts to save the lives of these premature infants.

OVER-THE-COUNTER MEDICATIONS

Over-the-counter medications are drugs, and there are only two that the pregnant woman can safely take: Tylenol and Robitussin, plain. Anything else should not be used during pregnancy, including adult-strength aspirin (325 mg). Aspirin interferes with platelet aggregation. (Platelets are small, colorless corpuscles in the blood that, clumping together, stop bleeding.) Because aspirin crosses the placenta, it can get to the brain of the growing fetus and cause intra-cranial bleeding. Women who have migraine headaches for which they take Fiorinal should switch to Fioricet because the latter contains acetaminophen instead of aspirin. Baby aspirin (78 mg), however, is often given to women who are at risk of losing a pregnancy.

For women who have arthritis and are pregnant, the only safe nonsteroidal anti-inflammatory drug is Disalcid, a prescription medicine. In aspirin, for which the chemical term is acetylsalicylic acid, it is the acetyl group that interferes with platelet aggregation.

This is absent in Disalcid, which is salicyl-salicylic acid, so it can be taken without fear that it will cause bleeding in the baby.

Colds. "I take Actifed." "I take Sudafed." "I take . . ." whatever, say women. I say, "Not while you're pregnant." When you have a cold, the small blood vessels in the nose are swollen and dilated, and these medications constrict them to take away the feeling of stuffiness. But they can also constrict the vessels of the placenta, which is highly vascular, and this constriction reduces oxygen flow to the fetus. If such medications cured the cold, I might say go ahead and take them, but since all they do is make you feel better temporarily, I believe the risks outweigh the benefits.

What I recommend for patients who are congested is a vaporizer, the old-time remedy used for croupy babies. Vicks makes a liquid called VapoSteam to be added to the water in the vaporizer; each droplet of steam then contains menthol and eucalyptus. These moisturize the mucous membranes, making you feel better without the potential of causing harm to the baby.

For a cough, Robitussin is okay during pregnancy even though it contains a small amount of alcohol. Nyquil, on the other hand, contains quite a bit of alcohol and should be avoided. The best thing for a cough and sore throat is a homemade cough syrup consisting of one-third lemon juice (from a real lemon, not a bottle), one-third honey, and one-third water. The honey soothes the throat, the lemon acts as an astringent for the phlegm, and the water keeps the mixture from sticking to your teeth.

Headaches. Two Tylenols are recommended in the case of a headache. Pregnant women have a tendency to go overboard in one direction or another, either taking everything or being too restrictive. "I have a headache, but I'll take half a Tylenol because I don't want to hurt the baby." Half a Tylenol is a drop in the bucket. The woman still has the headache, and she calls me. "Did you take two tablets? No? Okay, you have to go back and read the directions, which say you can take two, even two Extra Strength Tylenol. Take them. Quickly." Don't take more than eight Tylenols in a 24-hour period, but do take the prescribed dosage.

As for Advil and Motrin, which are ibuprofen, these are not recommended in pregnancy because there are no clinical trials as yet demonstrating their safety. If really needed, Advil can be used, but it is preferable to stick with Tylenol or Tylenol with codeine because these have been proven to be safe.

Vitamins. Prenatal multivitamin pills are prescribed for pregnant women and should be taken faithfully but not used as a substitute for a well-balanced diet. If you are not pregnant but thinking of becoming so, you should be taking folic acid. Spina bifida and other kinds of open neural tube defects—in which the vertebrae fail to form completely and part of the spinal cord is exposed—occur significantly more often in the babies of women whose diets are deficient in folic acid. A study done in the United Kingdom of women who had had a child with spina bifida showed that in subsequent pregnancies, the women given folic acid had normal children, while those whose diet was not supplemented with folic acid tended to have a second child with spina bifida. The recommendation is that if you are a woman of childbearing age, that is, between 15 and 44, you should have a daily folic acid intake of 0.4 milligrams. In order to ensure this intake in the average diet, the FDA has recently issued a regulation requiring folic acid to be added to enriched breads, flours, rice, pasta, and other grains. An adequate intake can also be ensured by eating plenty of raw, green, leafy vegetables like spinach and mustard greens, plus citrus fruits.

If you are already a vitamin aficionado and are taking lots of A, E, B-complex, or some other favorite, do not continue to do so without the advice of your obstetrician or a qualified nutritionist. Vitamins are not innocuous. A recent study, for example, showed that all too many babies were being born with birth defects because their mothers were taking high doses of vitamin A. The vitamins you take when pregnant have to be balanced and quantified.

X-RAYS AND MICROWAVES

When a pregnant woman is told to have a chest X-ray, the first thought that pops into her mind is a mushroom cloud and Hiroshima or Chernobyl. "X-ray, oh, my God, my baby's going to be . . ." No, it isn't. It takes an enormous amount of radiation to cause malformation, on the order of 25 rads (radiation absorbed dosage), and the average diagnostic dose is measured in millirads—a millirad is one-thousandth of a rad. Radiation is a very rare cause of birth defects and would only be a concern for somebody for whom radiation is an occupational hazard, such as workers in dental offices or radiology labs.

But radiation is an emotionally charged word and it is hard to extirpate the fear of it. I get calls from interns asking if they dare schedule a sophisticated type of scan for a pregnant woman. "How old is the fetus?" I ask. "Thirty-two weeks? Go right ahead." It is during the first 12 weeks that brain, liver, lungs, heart, and all the other organs are being formed. That is when birth defects get set in place; after that the fetus is simply enlarging on the basic structure.

Actually, this period is not even the whole of the first 12 weeks. From the moment of conception until 17 days later, whatever is done either will not affect the conceptus or it will totally abort it because the cells do not even know what they want to be yet. If something happens, either all the cells go away or they all go right on to be a limb or a liver or whatever. When something like the thalidomide babies happens, it is because the drug was taken 21 to 40 days after conception. This is not to say that after three months, you can go back to smoking, wine-drinking, or whatever; these will affect the *development* of the baby even though the basic structure is now in place.

According to the Centers for Disease Control (CDC), "Ionizing radiation is a wave or particle with sufficient energy to break bonds and create ions capable of causing tissue damage, and thus birth defects." Only X-rays and gamma rays have this degree of energy. Microwaves, by virtue of their lower energy, cannot produce ionization. Neither can magnetic resonance imaging (MRIs). Ultrasound is a mechanical as opposed to an electromagnetic wave, so it too is incapable of producing ionization. X-rays, then, are the only threat to the fetus, but not in the dosages customarily used, and if the abdomen is shielded with a lead apron, it becomes a moot point anyway.

ENVIRONMENTAL HAZARDS

A woman came to her gynecologist with anemia and irregular bleeding, and the gynecologist hospitalized her. Then another woman entered the hospital with the same symptoms. It happened that one nurse took care of both of them, and she asked the second patient what she did for a living. "I put tennis ball halves together," the patient said. The nurse then went to the first patient and asked her what she did for a living. "I work in a factory where I glue tennis balls." In this fashion was it discovered that the resin used in the factory affected the health of the women working there.

Women cannot count on management to protect them. They have to use common sense, most particularly if they are pregnant. They have to stand up and say, "I'm not taking a chance with my unborn child." How can you know if you are taking a chance? If you don't feel well, if you go home nauseated, your liver is working hard to cleanse you of toxins. But it cannot do everything, and you have to get out of the environment that is causing the reactions. Don't stick around, saying to yourself, "If this baby turns out to be defective, I am going to sue the company." Get out of there. It is better to be proactive than reactive.

MORNING SICKNESS

I am here to testify that morning sickness is the worst. I don't know who named it that—it must have been a man—because morning sickness can last all day. People say dismissively, "Oh, it's just morning sickness," and you agree. Until you get it; then you wish you were dead. You feel like you want to vomit but everything is stuck in your throat and you can't because there is nothing there. Your stomach is upset, and you want to heave and heave and heave, and you're sweating and retching as though you've swallowed a poisoned canary. It is not like a cold, not like the flu; it is far worse.

It may come in the morning and then go away, or it may last for the entire day, day after day. It may come when you are six weeks pregnant, or three, or ten, but most commonly it comes after eight weeks. It is supposed to last only until the end of the first trimester, which is 12 or 13 weeks. But four weeks of morning sickness is equivalent to four weeks of Chinese water torture. You are not fit company for man or beast.

The treatment for morning sickness used to be Bendectin, which contained vitamin B_6 and an antihistamine. But because morning sickness comes in the first trimester of pregnancy and that is when the baby's organs are being formed, Bendectin began to be blamed for any and all birth defects. The manufacturer could not afford the ensuing litigation and took the medication off the market. Now, to ease the nausea, all that pregnant women can turn to are crackers and ginger ale or cola drinks. Many women cannot eat at all because they vomit the food immediately. Drinking Emetrol, a high-dose carbohydrate liquid, is recommended to control the emesis, but some women toss that up too.

An occasional woman gets to the point where she cannot keep even water down and has to be hospitalized for hyperemesis gravidarum, an extreme form of morning sickness. She may require hyperalimentation in which nutrients are administered intravenously in order to correct the electrolyte imbalance and to give the mother needed nutrients lost in the constant vomiting. Just at the time in a woman's life when she is supposed to be so happy, it can all be ghastly and awful. With luck, the morning sickness ends at 12 or 13 weeks, but for two to five percent of women it is a nightmare that continues throughout pregnancy.

For unknown reasons, vitamin B6 can be effective in dealing with the nausea, but it has to be given by injection because pills are vomited. Some practitioners attempt to make their own "Bendectin" by prescribing vitamin B6 and a sleeping medication like Unisom, which contains an antihistamine. The *Physicians' Desk Reference* vetoes the practice for fear that it will give rise to lawsuits if babies are not normal, but an individual doctor may say, "She was so bad, I had to do something. Let's just hope that nothing happens."

As for the cause of morning sickness, it is thought to be an increase in hCG, the pregnancy hormone. The cliche is: "You're having morning sickness? Great! The more hCG you have, the more the placenta is really growing, and that's good." However, you may not find that very consoling when you are clinging to the porcelain steering wheel. Some women, perhaps because of low levels of hCG, do not suffer from morning sickness, while women who are carrying twins are particularly afflicted because of high levels of hCG. After the twelfth week of pregnancy, the level of hCG starts to stabilize, and that is when morning sickness usually ends.

VAGINAL BLEEDING

Implantation Bleeding. When the fertilized egg begins to burrow into the endometrial lining, disrupting some of the blood circulation, a harmless event called implantation bleeding may occur. However, it does not always happen, so it is unwise to dismiss vaginal bleeding. Women tend to say, "Oh, my sister had that. She says it's just implantation bleeding and it's okay." But it may not be. It may indicate an ectopic pregnancy or an impending miscarriage.

Implantation bleeding usually comes about two weeks after conception, so the woman may think it is her period. When she misses her next period and realizes that she is pregnant, she will answer her obstetrician's question about the date of her last period by giving the date of the implantation bleeding. A good obstetrician will ask, "Was that a normal period? Was it the same amount of bleeding as usual and was the duration the same?" If the woman answers, "Well, no, it was lighter than normal and it only lasted two days," the obstetrician knows that the patient is further along in her pregnancy than was first thought.

Ectopic Pregnancy. An ectopic pregnancy occurs when the fertilized conceptus becomes stuck in the fallopian tube, which can happen in women with tubal disease. The conceptus undergoes the same cell division in the tube as it would in the uterus, and as it increases in size, it ruptures the tube, causing bleeding and creating a medical emergency.

Hemorrhage previously accounted for the greatest number of maternal deaths, but it is now in second place behind thromboembolic causes, that is, blood clots in the lungs or brain. Nevertheless, hemorrhage remains a formidable enemy, and statistics show that when a woman dies from hemorrhage, the cause is usually a ruptured ectopic pregnancy. Thus, bleeding early in pregnancy or even at a time when the woman does not realize she is pregnant is to be taken seriously, never dismissed as, "Well, it's my period" or "It's nothing. Don't worry about it."

Miscarriage. Early in pregnancy, before the twelfth week, any bleeding may signal the beginning of the loss of the pregnancy. Ultrasound testing will help to distinguish a miscarriage from an ectopic pregnancy. For unknown reasons, about half of all pregnant women have some bleeding, and half of that half will go on to miscarry. That is, *one-fourth* of all pregnant women miscarry before the twelfth week.

We have no way of telling which half a particular pregnant woman will be in. When a patient calls me in a panic—"I'm bleeding! I'm spotting!"—I cannot tell her whether she is in the fifty percent who will miscarry or the fifty percent who will go on to have a healthy, full-term baby. All I can say is that she must go to bed and stay there until the bleeding stops. Often, with bed rest there is no further problem. But in some patients the bleeding continues, soaking one pad, then another; cramps set in; and the patient requires medical attention because a miscarriage may be on the way.

If there is only light bleeding or spotting, patients may demand, "Why don't you do something?"

"I cannot because I'm not in charge here. Nature is."

We do not know the reason behind the bleeding, and once it starts, we can only wait to see if nature will be kind and the bleeding will be self-limiting. If it is not, if it proceeds on to a miscarriage and the uterus expels the fetus, we as obstetricians are there to make sure the mother does not hemorrhage or become infected and that part of the products of conception do not remain behind in the uterus. We are only the cleanup squad; nature calls the shots.

If the bleeding at this early gestational age is less than a pad an hour, simple bed rest is prescribed, but if an external pad is soaked in an hour, the woman needs to be in the hospital. If an ultrasound examination shows that the little fetal heart is beating, and if the cervix is not dilated, we know that so far the baby is still okay and we can hope that maybe the placenta is just having a bad day and that things will go on to correct themselves.

When it does not work out that way, the patient miscarries, and she often asks what she did wrong. I say, "You didn't do anything wrong. This is your body's way of saying this wasn't a one hundred percent perfect baby. Either the baby or the placenta wasn't healthy and didn't click off the things the body expects it to click off by eight weeks. If it doesn't click them off, the pregnancy is shut down and you miscarry."

One of my patients had a miscarriage, and she and her husband asked, "What could it be? We wanted this baby so much." The husband listened carefully as I said that the body has its own way of deciding whether a pregnancy should go on. Then he suddenly commented, "It's like making flapjacks, isn't it? The first one is not the way you want it to be, so you throw it away. After that, the rest turn out okay."

"Right!" I said, and from then on I have used that analogy with my patients. It eases the patient's fear that somehow she did something to cause the miscarriage, and it also helps her to feel less sad. I tell the patient, "It's best your body was vigilant and turned the flow across the placenta off because if your body is asleep at the switch and does not shut down a defective pregnancy, that is when we discover at 25 or 36 weeks that this is a baby with anomalies and the real trouble begins."

A woman's first and second miscarriages occurring in the first trimester are not necessarily meaningful, but if it happens a third time, the products of conception should be sent to a pathology laboratory for evaluation, and the blood of the mother and father should be tested to make sure neither has a balanced translocation of his or her chromosomes. That sounds complicated, but imagine two whole pies; an equal size slice is cut from each one and exchanged. They are still two whole pies, but something is different about them. In the same way, a parent may have what appears to his or her own body to be perfectly arranged chromosomes but one in the series may be switched with another in a balanced translocation. This is no problem until that person mates with another with the same translocation and the chromosomes are halved. Then there is trouble with the offspring.

When a miscarriage occurs, the patient may say, "I passed it all, I think, in the toilet," in which event we wait to see if the uterus is going to continue to bleed. The uterus wants to be clean; it will eject anything that is not supposed to be in there, so if it keeps on bleeding, we know that some material has been retained and we must go in and empty out the uterus with what is called a completion D and C.

In addition to the possibility of hemorrhage, it is important to notify your doctor about bleeding because you may be Rh negative and need to be given RhoGAM immediately (see chapter 9). Without it, you develop antibodies and your next pregnancy will not be as smooth as it might have been.

Bleeding Late in Pregnancy. Vaginal bleeding in the last trimester of pregnancy is fraught with concern because the baby at a pound or two is a real baby and we want, if at all possible, to save it. The bleeding may happen because the placenta has prematurely separated from its base or because it implanted close to the cervix when it should have implanted high up at the top of the uterus. Close to the cervix, it may disrupt the blood vessels there and the mother starts to bleed. This condition is called placenta previa and is dealt with initially by bed rest with the hope that the bleeding will subside. The mother is hospitalized until she approaches term. At about 36 weeks, a month before her due date, amniocentesis is done to gauge the development of the fetal lungs. If they are sufficiently mature, the baby is then delivered by cesarean section.

In placenta previa the bleeding is usually painless. In abruptio placentae, on the other hand, the presentation is painful bleeding. Abruptio placentae is the premature separation from the wall of the uterus of a normally implanted placenta, and it occurs most commonly in women with high blood pressure and in women who smoke. Crack cocaine users also have a very high incidence of abruptio placentae. Trauma, as in car accidents or a blow to the abdomen in domestic violence, is another cause of the placenta being ripped off its base. One patient of mine fell off a ladder while trying to paint the baby's room because "my husband didn't want to do it." She started having cramps and pain and bleeding and was rushed to the hospital. The baby had to be delivered immediately because its support mechanism—the placenta—had been lost.

Home accidents in general are to be guarded against with the greatest care. There is nothing wrong with tub baths for a pregnant woman—except the danger of falling in the tub. Help getting in and out of the tub is recommended. Equal care should be exercised in the shower; a rubber mat is a good idea to prevent slips. The pregnant woman has to be careful about tripping on area rugs and the edges of carpets, and particularly careful about falling down stairs.

In the movies a woman falls off a horse and is told she cannot have any more babies. But that is the movies; nothing about a fall off a horse prevents a woman from having babies—unless she fractures her pelvis, but even then she can have babies by cesarean section. The only way you can have a uterus and not have babies is if the uterus becomes infected.

BED REST

One reads in novels about women having to stay in bed throughout their pregnancies, but this is true only if it is a multifetal gestation, that is, triplets or quadruplets, and even then the mother can get up and walk around a little. The other indication for bed rest is an incompetent cervix. The weight of a pregnancy can be too much for a cervix that has been weakened by previous pregnancies. Without labor contractions, without forewarning, the cervix opens up and lets everything fall out at 20 weeks or 23 weeks and the baby is lost.

When this is a possibility because of a previous loss after 20 weeks of pregnancy, at 14 weeks into the next pregnancy the obstetrician puts a stitch like a purse string in the cervix to draw it closed, and the woman is asked to stay home and lie in bed for the remainder of the pregnancy. These days the most frequent objection is "I can't do that. I have to work," so a lot of women are walking around with cerclages, which is what the procedure is called. Some get away with it; some do not.

MULTIPLE GESTATIONS

There are two mechanisms that cause multiple gestations. Two, three, or more eggs may be released, and each one may be fertilized; or a single egg may divide one or more times. The latter, the cleavage of a single egg, occurs once in 250 pregnancies and results in identical twins. Fraternal twins, on the other hand, come from separate eggs. Just as there can be double yolks in a hen's egg, some women are double, or even triple, ovulators. Two or three eggs are spewed out, Dad's sperm comes in and hits them all, and twins or triplets result.

If the pregnancy is a multifetal gestation, as determined by ultrasound, the mother has to be warned that one or more fetuses may not survive. The human female, unlike frogs or dogs, is basically designed to have one child at a time. One uterus, one child, so if two are in there, either the twins will jockey for position, each attempting to get a preferential blood flow, or both will grow but be small.

In a twin pregnancy, serial ultrasound examinations are carried out every three to four weeks to follow the growth of the fetuses. If one is outstripping the other but both are previable—that is, neither can survive outside the womb—all the obstetrician can do is wait; no intervention is possible. But if one of the twins being followed has always been smaller, and six weeks before the due date the difference in size has greatly increased, then the concern is: why the discordant growth? Each fetus is supposedly in its own little sac with its own placental circulation. Or is that not true? Is one placenta feeding and nurturing both twins? If the difference between the fetuses started out at 10 percent, then became 15 percent, at 20 weeks 25 percent, now at 34 weeks there is a 30 percent difference—one baby is two and a half pounds and distressed, the other four pounds—I as an obstetrician would say we have to go in; we have to deliver these twins despite the likelihood of lung immaturity and respiratory distress syndrome because whatever process is going on will continue and kill off the smaller twin.

Before there was ultrasound, we had no idea how many fetuses were in the womb. When the woman delivered, she delivered one baby, but that child could have started out as three and two died on the way or two and one died on the way. With ultrasound, and especially with CVS (see chapter 8), we see multiple gestations all the time. We see triplets and quadruplets early in pregnancy, but three weeks down the line, without any intervention, two of them are gone. One or more simply withers away and is absorbed. The pregnancy can start as twins and before you know it, there is just a singleton because one has usurped all the nutrients, has laid claim to a preferential blood flow; nature has selected one over the other. However, it is not like a miscarriage; the lost fetus is not expelled. It calcifies; what is left can turn to rock. Or it can become what is called fetal papyraceous, that is, like paper, mummified. In either event, it usually comes out with the afterbirth. This phenomenon is known as "the vanishing twin syndrome."

At the delivery of a singleton, if you know that twins were there originally, you try to see what happened to the fetus because the patient may be a double ovulator and at risk for carrying twins again. Because it is desirable to gather as much information as possible, the placenta should be sent to a pathology laboratory for an in-depth analysis of what went wrong.

Selective Reduction. Some couples who have heard about selective reduction (see chapter 7) seek counseling when they learn that the mother is carrying natural triplets or quadruplets. The mother has not had any sort of ovulation induction medication; it has just happened that she has released three eggs and the father has fertilized them. The couple wonders if the number should be reduced to twins. This involves bioethical issues, but in any event I am inclined to advise against it because injecting potassium chloride into the heart of one of the fetuses is an invasive procedure and I am not in favor of any invasive procedure, no matter how apparently safe. And nature itself may intervene to reduce the number.

POINTS TO REMEMBER

- Home pregnancy tests do not differentiate between a normal and an ectopic pregnancy. If your test is positive, see a doctor promptly.
- Pregnancy is dated from the first day of the last period and is calculated in weeks, not months.
- Tell no one but your husband that you are pregnant until the 26th week.
- One-fourth of all pregnancies end in miscarriage.
- Excessive weight gain is the single most important source of complications in pregnancy. Remember that you are not eating for two but one and a twentieth. Hold total weight gain to 24 to 26 pounds.
- Drink eight glasses of water and a quart of skim milk a day. Dehydration can cause premature labor.
- No smoking and no alcohol of any kind during pregnancy.
- Walking half an hour a day in the open air is the best exercise during pregnancy.
- Carefully consider your working conditions and hours. Insufficient rest is a primary cause of premature labor.
- The only safe over-the-counter medications during pregnancy are Tylenol and Robitussin, plain. Aspirin should be avoided.
- Diagnostic X-rays are not hazardous to the fetus after the first 12 weeks.
- Toxic work environments are to be avoided.
- Morning sickness is most common between the eighth and twelfth weeks. There is no effective treatment for it.
- Vaginal bleeding in pregnancy requires immediate medical attention.
- In multiple gestations—twins, triplets, or quadruplets—nature may intervene to reduce the number.

6

I'M PREGNANT—
AND I DON'T WANT TO BE

❧

FIRST TRIMESTER ABORTION • MENSTRUAL EXTRACTION • D AND C • SECOND TRIMESTER ABORTION • DRUG ABORTION • RU-486 • COMPARISON OF RISK •

"You have a positive pregnancy test, and your uterus is eight weeks' size."

I have said that many a time in my office and witnessed reactions ranging from great happiness to fear to sadness. When a patient is upset by the news that she is pregnant, the reason may be that a baby will interfere with her education or her work, or the family cannot afford another child; or she may not be in a stable relationship and feels that she cannot accept the responsibility of being a single parent. This is the point at which a woman must make up her mind whether or not to continue the pregnancy, and it is she who must live with the consequences of that decision. No politician, no priest, not even her own mother can or should make the decision for her. Nor can an obstetrician or gynecologist; we are simply available to make the decision less threatening to her life, whether it is to continue the pregnancy or end it.

In any one year, three percent of American women between the ages of 15 and 44 have an abortion, that is, three out of every one hundred women of reproductive age. There is a general perception that abortion is common and increasing, but in fact the incidence has gone down. In 1982 there were 1,573,900 abortions in the United States; in 1992 there were 1,529,000. There is an equally common perception that it is usually teenagers who terminate a pregnancy, but abortion is frequent among women who already have two or three children. The highest rate is among women aged 20 to 24, the second highest is among women aged 25 to 29.

No particular evidence suggests that women are abusing the right to abortion. But centuries of evidence exist to show that women will have abortions no matter what societal, legal, or moral strictures are put in their way. All the legislation in the world is not going to stop the woman who is met with a positive pregnancy test if she already has all the children she wants or can take care of, or her husband has just left her, or she will be in danger of losing her livelihood. If you have seen, as I did in the days before *Roe v. Wade*, wards full of women deadly ill because of septic or botched abortions, you will not believe that the clock should be turned back and abortion once again be made illegal.

FIRST TRIMESTER ABORTION

To keep the record straight, there are two kinds of abortion: spontaneous and induced. A miscarriage in early pregnancy is a spontaneous abortion; an induced abortion is a deliberately interrupted pregnancy.

Menstrual Extraction. If it is very early in the pregnancy, at about five weeks' gestation, menstrual extraction can be used to end the pregnancy. Extraction is basically no different from an endometrial biopsy in that an instrument is introduced into the uterus to aspirate, that is, suction out, the conceptus.

D and C. If the gestation period has gone beyond five weeks, the patient requires a D and C—the same dilatation and curettage used in the presence of irregular bleeding or suspected polyp, performed with the same instruments, plus a vacuum aspirator, which sucks out the products of conception under negative pressure. The products of conception go into a receptacle in the machine and are sent to a laboratory for identification of the fetus and placenta. This procedure is important because if the uterus has been emptied out by aspiration but the laboratory finds none of the signs of pregnancy, the pregnancy may be in the patient's fallopian tube or ovary or abdomen and the uterus is responding to it with the hormonal changes of pregnancy just as though it is in its proper place. Anti-abortion activists make the process sound dreadful, saying, "The baby's parts are cut up," but it is necessary to identify what has been aspirated in order to make certain that the pregnancy is not ectopic.

The earlier the D and C is done, the less bleeding, the less trauma, and the fewer complications there are. The procedure can be done under local anesthesia, but to my mind that is a brutal way to go about it. Dilatation of the cervix is painful, but even worse is the sucking sound of the vacuum. Women who are awake and hear it may have nightmares for years afterwards, and many have depressive episodes. Even though the anesthesiologist may argue that it is less risky to use local or epidural anesthesia, if one takes the whole patient into account, the humane approach is to put the patient to sleep and have her wake up in the recovery room. Women should be aware that they do have an option and insist upon general anesthesia or heavy sedation if they feel that it will make the abortion less emotionally traumatic.

Patients usually do not lose much blood with a D and C, and since it is a sterile procedure, the infection rate is very low and child-bearing at a later date is not affected. In Russia until recently, because the Pill and the diaphragm were not widely available, abortions were the accepted means of family planning, and many women had a dozen or more abortions without ill effect. I am often asked by women who have had one or two abortions whether their cervix is stable enough to support a pregnancy. The answer is yes. After an abortion the cervix returns to its nonpregnant state as long as there has been no infection or laceration. Should the woman desire to become pregnant, however, she should wait for at least two cycles after an induced or spontaneous abortion in order to allow everything to stabilize.

The downside of abortions, and of D and Cs in general, is that it is easy to scrape the uterus too deeply, causing what is known as Asherman's syndrome. If the curettage is too vigorous, the layers of the uterine lining will not regenerate and the patient will not have her period. Failure to have a period after a D and C should send the patient back to her doctor because she needs to be on medication to build the layer back up again.

Following an abortion, the despondency and sense of bereavement can be just as acute as it is with a miscarriage. Women do what they feel is best for their families and their lives, but it is never an easy decision, and for them to be judged by people who are not in their situation is, I feel, unfair. Although I myself do not perform abortions, I will fight for a woman's right to have one. And if it really came down to it, if I were the last obstetrician in the world and I knew the woman really needed to have a termination, I guess I would do it. But my principles are mine, and neither I nor anyone else can get inside the head of another person. I feel the decision is between a woman and her Creator, and it calls for no interference from anyone else.

Once upon a time not so long ago, women used coat hangers and scissors and potassium permanganate and went to butchers in back rooms, whatever it took to get an abortion. After *Roe v. Wade*, the medical community said, all right, we know what has been happening in the past. Now, how can we make it so that *two* people are not going to be dead—the mother as well as the unborn fetus—and that is when safe and legal abortions became available.

The Right-to-Life people picket and protest, but when they get through with their stint on the sidewalk in front of the clinic, they go have their cup of coffee and Danish, while the lady who is pregnant is still pregnant. What I would like to have the Pro-Life people do is to put their names on a list. The two or three million or more people in this country who are Pro-Life could then constitute a national Pro-Life bank, and the woman who becomes pregnant but cannot afford to have a baby, emotionally or economically, could say, "You're at the top of the list. I am going to turn the baby over to you." By rights, the Pro-Lifer should answer, "Fine. I will raise your child." But the old man or the middle-aged woman who has been picketing does not say that, so the woman goes to the next person on the list. And so on. How many names does she go through before she finds someone willing to take the child? Hundreds? Thousands? All of them? It is easy to march for a cause, to argue on behalf of a theoretical child, but to take responsibility for an actual child can be quite a different matter.

SECOND TRIMESTER ABORTION

The second trimester begins at about 13 weeks and ends at 26 to 28 weeks. State laws in general allow abortions up to 26 or 28 weeks, but few hospitals permit it beyond 22 weeks. Some set the cutoff time at 20 or 21 weeks, which is why it is important for women undergoing prenatal diagnosis, that is, amniocentesis, in the second trimester to find out how long it is going to take to get the results. If the baby has anomalies but this is not known until after the cutoff date, abortion is not permitted unless the anomalies are such as to be incompatible with life.

As described in connection with prenatal testing (Chapter 8), a second trimester termination of pregnancy means going through labor and places the mother at higher risk of hemorrhage, infection, and the complication of a retained placenta. But the increased risk is not the only reason to avoid a second trimester abortion if at all possible; it is a harrowing experience to go through the pain of labor only to deliver a dead child.

DRUG ABORTION

A 1995 report in the *New England Journal of Medicine* described the successful trial of two FDA-approved drugs used in combination to bring about an abortion: an abortifacient, methotrexate, which kills the fetus, and a prostaglandin-type drug (misoprostol), which causes contractions. In the small number of patients in the trial, abortion was induced in 95 percent, which suggests that the surgical approach to abortion may soon be a thing of the past.

The methotrexate is administered by a series of intramuscular injections in doses based on the patient's weight. After these take effect, the patient is given prostaglandin pills to take or suppositories that she inserts herself. These drugs are not available over the counter, but the termination does take place in the privacy of the patient's own home, which is psychologically easier than having to go to a clinic. The patient is made aware of the signs of an incomplete abortion, so that she knows to return for a D and C should that be necessary.

RU-486

Mifepristone (RU-486) is poised for FDA approval. It is a potent antiprogesterone steroid. A single dose (600 mg), when taken by mouth no later than 49 days after the last menstrual period, results in loss of a documented pregnancy in 90 percent of patients.

How this antiprogesterone works is not known, but it is thought to compete with progesterone for receptor sites in the uterus, resulting in the sloughing off of the uterine lining. In addition, the drug's prostaglandin-stimulating effects simultaneously cause the uterus to contract. Early clinical trials have suggested that the sooner RU-486 is used, the more effective it is in achieving pregnancy loss.

The most serious side-effect of RU-486 is prolonged bleeding (up to 16 days). Compared with the surgical approach for early termination of pregnancy, suction currettage, RU-486 is less effective (90 percent versus 99 percent), slower (days versus minutes), and is associated with greater blood loss. However, it offers privacy for the patient and does not require an injection or surgery.

Unfortunately, RU-486 has become embroiled in the political firestorm surrounding abortion. Its availability will depend on whether the FDA ultimately approves it for use in this country.

COMPARISON OF RISK

The risk of a woman's dying is eleven to sixteen times greater if she delivers a baby at term than if she has a termination of pregnancy. Shocking, but true. In 1972, before *Roe v. Wade*, the mortality rate in women having an abortion was 4.1 per 100,000, while the maternal mortality rate was 18.9 per 100,000. Both figures have gone down since then—in 1987 the abortion mortality rate was 0.4, with the maternal mortality rate at 6.6—but it still is safer to have an abortion than to have a baby. The lay public tends to believe just the opposite, assuming that no one dies in childbirth anymore and that abortion with all those instruments invading the body is really dangerous, but this is simply not so. There is less than one death for every 500,000 abortions performed at eight weeks or less, compared to thirty deaths as a result of continued pregnancy and its complications.

POINTS TO REMEMBER

- Abortion performed in the first trimester, 0 to 12 weeks, is the safest and easiest.

- Almost 99 percent of first trimester abortions are carried out by means of a D and C.
- Abortion under general anesthesia is less traumatic than under local or epidural anesthesia.
- There is a less than one percent risk of serious complications from abortion.

7

I'M NOT PREGNANT—
AND I WANT TO BE

෨෧

THE MALE FACTORS • THE FEMALE FACTORS • FALLOPIAN
TUBES • OVULATION • UTERINE AND CERVICAL FACTORS •
ASSISTED TECHNOLOGIES • IN VITRO FERTILIZATION •
GAMETE INTRAFALLOPIAN TRANSFER • EMOTIONAL AND
FINANCIAL COST • BIRTH DEFECTS •

Rather than being concerned with how to prevent pregnancy, some number of women, particularly older women, have the opposite problem: They wish to conceive and cannot. I described earlier how eggs are present in the female from the time she is in her mother's womb, which means that when a woman is 30 years old, the eggs, too, are 30 years old and tend to be less fertile. There are also fewer of them, and thus a woman of that age and older may have difficulty becoming pregnant. However, even when age is not a factor, a couple may have trouble conceiving a child.

Infertility is defined as the inability to become pregnant after one year of unprotected intercourse. This condition affects approximately 15 percent of couples in the United States. The major problem areas in cases of infertility are the male factor (35 to 40%) and in the female, the fallopian tubes (20 to 25%), the ovaries (15 to 20%), the uterus or cervix (5 to 15%).

THE MALE FACTORS

People tend to assume, when the question of infertility comes up, that the trouble is with the wife, but that is probably true in only about 50 percent of cases. If the wife is seen by a gynecologist and it is determined that she is ovulating each month, then attention should turn to the husband with respect to sperm count, sperm motility, and whether or not he may have what is called a varicocele, a varicose condition of the veins in the scrotal area that precludes the sperm's maturing sufficiently to fertilize an egg. This latter is a correctable condition, and after it is remedied, there may be no further problem with the wife's becoming pregnant.

In an examination of the husband, the history should include an inquiry about sports injuries (especially testicular trauma); mumps; and heat, radiation, or toxin exposure. Use of drugs such as marijuana or of anabolic steroids (testosterone) for body-building is of particular concern.

Laboratory studies should include a semen analysis, evaluation for the presence of sperm antibodies, and a sperm penetration test. The semen analysis is carried out after two to three days of abstinence from intercourse. Two hours after ejaculation, when the semen is examined, the amount of semen should be in the range of less than a teaspoonful to half a tablespoon (2 to 6 ml), with at least twenty million sperm per milliliter; 60 percent of them should have a normal shape, and at least 50 percent of them should be motile. If clumping of the sperm is observed, sperm antibody tests are performed in order to identify the presence of antibodies directly attached to the sperm. The functioning of the sperm is analyzed by observing their ability to penetrate hamster eggs, on the theory that if a human sperm can penetrate a hamster egg, it can penetrate a human egg.

If the husband's sperm count is sufficient and the wife is ovulating, the advice I give patients is not to have intercourse too frequently. Sometimes the woman is so obsessed with wanting to become pregnant that the demands she makes on her partner can lead to male performance problems. The wife, checking her ovulometer, an over-the-counter device that detects when the ovary is just about to release an egg, calls her husband at the office and says excitedly, "It's time, it's time, it's time," and he is expected to hurry home and perform on cue. For some men this is a turnoff. If the relationship begins to suffer, a wise woman will pull back at this point and ask herself whether it might not be better to go about the attempt to get pregnant in more relaxed fashion.

Although an egg is only fertilizable for 24 hours, the sperm can last for four or five days, so there is not that much rush for the husband to get home. If the number and motility and shape of the sperm are normal and an egg is being ovulated, there is no reason for exaggerated concern about timing. Intercourse three times a week, four times at most— every other night but not more than once a night— should result in a pregnancy. More frequent intercourse simply lowers the husband's sperm count, and, anyway, there is only so much the poor man can go through before, psychologically, it becomes a job. The guy who is 32 or 42 is not the same fellow he was when he was 16 and in the back seat of a Chevy. Now he is saying, "Honey, is this over yet?" If and when it is and his wife is pregnant, all he wants is a time-out, a cooling off period; don't mention sex, he doesn't want to hear about it. If—God forbid—there is a miscarriage, the expression on the husband's face suggests the world has come to an end: "Do I have to go through this all over again?"

As well as making life difficult for her husband, the overly determined wife may be making trouble for herself. It has been my observation that, just as a watched pot does not boil, a stressed ovary does not ovulate. The more a woman frets about becoming pregnant, the higher the stress level and the less likely she is to conceive. My advice all around is: Relax, take it easy, just do what comes naturally.

THE FEMALE FACTORS

As a general rule, 85 percent of women having unprotected intercourse will become pregnant, if not immediately, at least within a year. The young woman who wishes to have a baby but fails to conceive after having unprotected intercourse three times a week for a year should seek professional advice from her gynecologist. If the woman is older than 35, she will perhaps do better not to let that much time go by; four to six months is long enough to wait before seeking an initial gynecologic evaluation.

Fallopian Tubes. To determine the cause of infertility, the gynecologist will explore several possibilities, beginning with whether the fallopian tubes are open to permit the passage of an egg. The patient's past history is usually more helpful than the physical examination in this regard. A history of pelvic inflammatory disease, sexually transmitted disease, or use of an IUD, even a history of a ruptured appendix, are valuable pieces of information.

Hysterosalpingogram (HSG). To evaluate the size and shape of the uterus and the patency of the fallopian tubes, an HSG may be done. This study requires an X-ray of the pelvis. Radiopaque dye (preferably water-based as it is safer than oil-based) is injected through the cervix into the uterus. If the fallopian tubes are normal, the dye is seen flowing through them, and conversely, any obstruction or abnormality will be shown impeding the flow. This HSG study does not require anesthesia, although it may cause moderate to severe pelvic discomfort or pain.

Laparoscopy. The presence of pelvic inflammatory disease or endometriosis can only be established by means of the operative technique of laparoscopy. Carbon dioxide, which minimizes the chance of injury to the bowel, is introduced through a narrow needle inserted just below the navel, and a scope with a fiberoptic light source is inserted into the abdomen. The entire pelvis is visualized through the scope, and if necessary, surgery is performed, using laser technology. If significant fallopian tube damage is seen, however, in vitro fertilization will probably be preferable to surgery.

Ovulation. The most common means used for confirming the release of an egg from an ovary is charting the basal body temperature. A rise in temperature of one-half to three-quarters of a degree signals the release. Other methods of identifying ovulation are the measurement of serum progesterone in midcycle or observing the disappearance of the large egg follicle on ultrasound.

Luteal Phase Defect. This occurs when the remnant of the follicle that has just released the egg, the corpus luteum, does not function properly and the progesterone level, which is usually very high at this stage, is low. Without the expected progesterone level, the uterine lining is poorly prepared for the fertilized egg to implant. This abnormality is identified by an in-office endometrial biopsy in which a sample of tissue is taken from the lining of the womb to see if it shows a less-than-expected stage of growth.

Anovulatory Cycles. If it is determined that there are cycles when no egg is being released, a hormonal evaluation is necessary. This includes a thyroid function test, a test for levels of prolactin (the hormone responsible for milk production), and tests to establish the levels of follicle-stimulating hormone (FSH) and luteinizing hormone (LH). (The latter two hormones are important for the regulation of ovarian function.)

After it has been documented that ovulation is not occurring, a nonsteroidal drug, Clomid (clomiphene citrate), taken orally, is usually prescribed. Clomid causes an increase in FSH and LH release, which leads to egg maturation and eventually ovulation. Treatment is usually begun on the fourth or fifth day of the menstrual cycle at the lowest dosage and is continued for five consecutive days. Ovulation should occur one week after the last pill is taken, but if it does not, the dosage is increased in subsequent cycles. After three or four cycles, if ovulation is still not taking place, an injection of the pregnancy hormone hCG is given at midcycle. If this treatment also fails, the patient is invited to begin treatment with Pergonal.

Pergonal is human menopausal gonadotropin hormone which is high in both FSH and LH. In contrast to Clomid, which is taken orally, an ampule of Pergonal must be injected daily. Because too many follicles may be stimulated to develop with this treatment, careful monitoring by means of sonograms and measurement of the body's estrogen level is necessary. If more than four follicles with eggs are developing, ovarian hyperstimulation syndrome can occur in which there is ovarian enlargement with abdominal bloating and discomfort accompanied by sudden weight gain. The ovaries leak fluid into the abdominal cavity, and the increase in abdominal fluid (ascites) can cause difficulty in breathing that can progress to a life-threatening situation.

When ovulation is stimulated by the administration of Clomid or Pergonal, more than one egg may be released, resulting in multiple gestations. The normal frequency of twins in the general population is one in 88 to 90 pregnancies, but this figure changes to one in 20 with Clomid; that is, instead of a one percent chance of twins, you have a five percent chance. With Pergonal, the probability increases to 20 percent. Most often the multiple gestation is twins, but triplets, quadruplets, and quintuplets are not rare.

An ultrasound examination done as early as five or six weeks into the pregnancy can determine if the gestation is multiple because each fetus will be in a separate sac and the sacs are visible. Wanting to know early in pregnancy how many fetuses are present is more than a matter of curiosity. The more fetuses there are, the lower are the chances of all, or even any, surviving. Selective reduction of the number of fetuses by injection of potassium chloride into the heart of one or more fetuses increases the chances that the remaining fetuses will survive to a more advanced age, but, as noted, the procedure is fraught with many bioethical issues.

Uterine and Cervical Factors. Again the woman's history is important. Previous uterine surgery, for example, a D and C, may have resulted in scarring of the lining of the uterus, or a cone biopsy of the cervix may have compromised mucus production, causing the appropriately elastic mucus not to be produced. Examining the uterine cavity by means of hysteroscopy, using carbon dioxide or a similar substance to separate the walls of the uterus, establishes the diagnosis. If a uterine septum (dividing wall), polyps, adhesions, or small myomas are present, they can be removed at the same time.

Postcoital Test. The purpose of this test is twofold: it evaluates both the sperm quality and the quantity and quality of the cervical mucus. Just before ovulation and several hours after sexual intercourse, mucus is collected from the cervix and placed on a slide, where it is examined for clarity, the presence of spinnbarkeit (stretchability), and the presence of motile sperm. If the mucus is of poor quality, oral estrogen may be prescribed or the patient may be offered intrauterine insemination.

ASSISTED TECHNOLOGIES

In 15 percent of infertile couples, no cause of infertility can be found. These couples may benefit from assisted reproductive technologies such as gamete intrafallopian transfer (GIFT), zygote intrafallopian transfer (ZIFT), or in vitro fertilization (IVF).

In Vitro Fertilization. The first IVF child was born in England in 1978. Since then, thousands of children have been born with the aid of this technology, which consists of stimulating ovulation, egg retrieval, egg fertilization, embryo transfer to the uterus, and implantation. Because skill and experience are essential to the successful carrying out of these steps, in vitro fertilization should only be conducted by a team headed by a Board-Certified obstetrician-gynecologist who specializes in reproductive endocrinology and has completed his or her fellowship training.

Ovulation Stimulation. Coaxing the eggs to mature involves the use of both gonadotropin-releasing hormone (GnRH) and Pergonal. The GnRH is given as an injection under the skin or in a nasal spray, while the Pergonal is administered by daily injections into a muscle, usually the buttock. The goal of ovulation stimulation is to achieve a "lead" follicle 17 millimeters in diameter, and at least three or four other follicles that measure 14 or 15 millimeters in diameter. When that has been achieved, a single dose of hCG, the pregnancy hormone, is given in order to trigger the final maturation of the follicles.

Egg Retrieval. Eggs, technically referred to as oocytes, are retrieved about 36 hours after the hCG injection has been administered. Using endovaginal ultrasound, the eggs are aspirated in rapid succession with a needle guided by the ultrasound picture.

I have known gynecologist-obstetricians who elected to go into reproductive endocrinology "because I want my nights off, Yvonne. You've got OB, you're up all night long." But with the complex techniques that have been developed, it turns out that they are working all hours of the day and night now, too. Pergonal shots have to be given at a certain hour, followed by hCG at a certain hour, followed by harvesting of the eggs at a certain hour. The infertility specialist may well be in the hospital at five o'clock in the morning if that is when the time is just right for the harvesting.

Egg Fertilization. After the eggs are identified under a microscope, they are covered by sperm in a Petri dish, which is a clear, covered, shallow dish. A day later, if fertilization has occurred, the eggs are transferred into the uterus. The transfer takes place approximately 48 hours after retrieval. Extra embryos may be frozen for transfer to the uterus at a future date. However, the success rate for cryopreservation is on the order of only 5 to 10 percent.

In the old days, which were not very long ago in this field, infertility specialists who carried out fertilization of eggs outside of the womb would put back eight fertilized eggs, hoping that four would take. Sometimes six took, which meant there were six fertilized embryos in the uterus, and because that was too many, the woman went on to lose all six of them. We obstetricians asked the infertility specialists not to put so many eggs back in. Four at the most, we suggested, if the procedure takes, there will only be one or two embryos and they will have a better chance of surviving.

If all four take, selective reduction may be used to reduce them to two, but they are never reduced to a singleton for fear of losing the entire pregnancy. With six, the reduction might be to three. But it has to be remembered that with triplets, three babies are growing in a womb designed for one child. Because the uterus is overextended, there is an increased chance of preterm labor, and the premature infants may have neurological deficits and growth problems

In experienced hands, the selective reduction procedure has a five to ten percent chance of causing loss of the total pregnancy.

Gamete Intrafallopian Transfer (GIFT). This is a technique used when the female has at least one normal fallopian tube. In a process similar to IVF, the retrieved eggs and the sperm are placed together in a transfer catheter instead of the Petri dish. The catheter is then gently introduced into the distal (most distant from the uterus) third of the fallopian tube, where fertilization normally takes place, and the egg and sperm are released. This is a more natural environment for fertilization than a Petri dish.

Transfer of a fertilized egg into the fallopian tube less than 48 hours after retrieval is called zygote intrafallopian transfer (ZIFT). Success rates for both GIFT and ZIFT are reported to be higher than for IVF. Ectopic pregnancies, however, occur in 5 percent of women having these procedures, while in the general population the frequency is 1.7 percent.

EMOTIONAL AND FINANCIAL COST

If a patient of mine of any age wants to become pregnant, I encourage her to go through the initial office procedures of determining ovulation and her partner's sperm count, and then perhaps a trial of Clomid. But if these simple steps fail, before referring her to an infertility specialist, I suggest that some reality testing is in order. Because I am not the woman's mother or husband, I can perhaps be useful in helping her to look at the situation with some objectivity.

Just as a practical matter, starting with an infertility specialist means embarking on a roller-coaster ride that may be hard to call a halt to. The specialist tries this, tries that, and at what point does the patient say enough is enough? We're not Americans for nothing. It's Pike's Peak or bust. The husband feels like he is playing for the Giants and has to make a touchdown. "Did you get your period?" he asks anxiously. He feels like he has succeeded or failed depending solely on whether his wife gets her period. The whole dynamic of the relationship changes. Where initially it was, "Okay, we'll give it a try, and if we have kids, we have them," now it becomes a matter of life or death.

Then there is the matter of the cost. In vitro fertilization costs five to seven thousand dollars a shot, and it may need to be done as many as six or seven times. If the husband and wife are in their 40s, well established, and able to afford the cost, there are nevertheless things to think about beyond getting a fertilized egg and having it become an embryo and then a fetus and then a newborn. Even at 20, pregnancy is not always a piece of cake, and at 40 or more it can be a difficult proposition indeed. Those 20 years put a lot of mileage on a body. Life's little nicks and pings and dents have taken their toll, and it can be a rough nine months. Then comes childbirth.

When comedienne Fanny Brice said that having a baby was like delivering a piano through the transom, she was not kidding. At 40 or 45 the transom does not have a lot of give to it, and many older women end up needing a cesarean section.

"So it happens," a patient may say. "But then the baby's there, and we're both fine, and we go home from the hospital." Except that now sleep deprivation begins. Because she is determined to go the whole nine yards, Mommy is breast-feeding. The husband who has been her friend, her companion, her confidante all these years is suddenly odd man out. Now a little person is there between two people who have been as close as yoked oxen, a little person with exhausting demands, like a 2:00 A.M. feeding. The husband says, "Gee, I wish I could take over and let you get some sleep, Honey, but I don't have breasts." And even if it isn't a question of feeding but of changing or soothing a fretful baby, he still can't get up when the baby cries because he has to be fresh for work the next morning. Mommy is the one repeatedly struggling out of a warm bed during the night.

"Be prepared," I tell my patients. "It's like going without sleep for a period of six to twelve weeks." In my experience, sleep deprivation is the most underrated, least recognized cause of postpartum depression. When older mothers come back for their six-week checkup, they often say, "I bit off more than I can chew and I'm just barely making it. I had no idea it would be so rough."

Babies do stop being babies eventually, but then they become two- and three-year-olds. At this age they are bundles of energy, and Mommy is now heading toward fifty. There is no way she is going to be able to keep up, so she goes back to work and hands over her paycheck for day care. Actually, she may not think it a bad trade, for she has found she does not enjoy gossiping on playground benches with mothers thirty years younger than herself. She is too far away from her own childhood to want to be a Cub Scout leader or chaperone the class trip to Washington. She feels out of place attending P.T.A. meetings with parents half her age. She is mortified when someone congratulates her on having a beautiful grandchild.

In a way, it *is* like having a grandchild rather than a child. The parents are already the people they will become. They will not grow and change along with their child. They arrived some time ago, and they are involved in their own lives. They prefer the theater to Little League games. They are into symphonies, not rap. They like resorts, not campgrounds. They go traveling and leave the child home. And the child wonders: Why did they have me if they don't want to be with me?

Is it because the child was a trophy? Did the woman awaken one morning with the feeling that she has done everything except have a baby? Did she tell herself that menopause is just around the corner, it's last-chance café, and along with the BMW and the condo at the ski resort, she has to have a child to prove she is successful?

A child is not an object. A child is a human being who needs love and nurturing and huge amounts of attention to thrive. That is why I sit down and talk with women who want to be mothers at 42 or 43—whether fertility is yet a concern or not. It is not just delayed child-bearing but delayed child-rearing that needs to be factored into the equation. When the child is 17, at the height of activity and involvement, the woman is 60, and the psychological wars she has to deal with with a teenager are exhausting; their interests are worlds apart. Her life is winding down; the child's is revving up.

I have often heard the child of older parents say, "I'm having kids as soon as I can because I do not want my children to be in the situation I was in. I love my parents—don't get me wrong—but they were never around. They didn't play with me. They didn't enjoy the same things I did."

As I say, I seldom try to discourage a woman from trying the initial steps of Clomid or Pergonal to become pregnant. But when it is a question of proceeding to the more sophisticated forms of infertility testing and treatment, I suggest it is time for some hard thinking about whether or not this is the best path to go down.

BIRTH DEFECTS

At a recent seminar, a pediatric geneticist spoke about teratology, the medical term for birth defects. *Terato-* is a combining form meaning "monster," and this doctor had seen such monsters as a cycloptic fetus, a baby with just one eye. He commented that infertility may be nature's way of saying, "Please do not pass on your genes." If cows are unable to conceive, he said, they are sent off to be slaughtered, but if humans are unable to conceive, they are sent to Virginia for in vitro fertilization. Eggs not really meant to procreate are artificially combined with sperm, a child is born with a gene pool that may be defective, and something that nature did not want to be perpetuated is being passed on.

If I suggest to a woman that the wisest thing may be to accept that motherhood is not her destiny, the answer is often, "Oh, you don't know, you don't understand. We want a baby, we want a child so bad."

"I know what you want," I answer. "But there is your plan, and there is God's plan, and it is probably best to let God's plan win. If you lost your right arm, you'd say, 'All right, I'll get a prosthesis. I'll learn to write with my left hand. I'll do the best I can.' It is the same with infertility. After a certain point it is best not to fight it but to play the cards you've been dealt and get on with your life. Accept where you are, put your love into building an even stronger relationship with your husband, and be a wonderful resource for your nieces and nephews and your friends' children."

Recently I was on a TV show with a physician who spoke of having utilized in vitro fertilization with women of 48 and 55, even a woman of 61. These were wealthy women married to younger men, but just because they could afford to have this procedure, it does not follow that they should have it, in my opinion. As I remarked on the program, "You know, someone once said that we have gained much knowledge but no wisdom." At the very least, I believe we should lay out the downside clearly and firmly before we set about outwitting nature on our patients' behalf.

POINTS TO REMEMBER

- Eighty-five percent of women having unprotected intercourse will become pregnant within a year. If pregnancy does not happen, a young woman should consult her gynecologist at the end of the year, an older woman after four to six months.

- If you are trying to become pregnant, do not have intercourse more than once a night three or four times a week.
- The more a woman frets about becoming pregnant, the higher the stress level and the less likely she is to conceive.
- Approximately 50 percent of instances of infertility in couples involve the male partner.
- The frequency of multiple gestations increases sharply with fertility-inducing measures.
- In vitro fertilization should be conducted by a team headed by a Board-Certified obstetrician-gynecologist who specializes in reproductive endocrinology and has completed fellowship training.
- After the initial procedures of determining ovulation and partner's sperm count and a trial of Clomid, evaluate the situation carefully before proceeding to the emotionally and financially costly step of in vitro fertilization.
- Any woman over 40 should carefully consider the long-term emotional and physical challenges of childbearing and child-rearing before having a baby.

III

CHILDBIRTH

❧

8

PRENATAL TESTING

୨୧

MATERNAL ALPHA-FETOPROTEIN • ULTRASOUND • AMNIO-
CENTESIS • CHORIONIC VILLUS SAMPLING • RISK FACTORS
IN CVS VERSUS AMNIOCENTESIS • GENETIC COUNSELING •
THE TERMINATION DECISION

Any prospective parent can request prenatal testing for purposes of determining whether the fetus is normal, and many do because they are reluctant to bring a child into the world who is unable to be a productive citizen in a society that values independence. By far the most common reason for prenatal diagnostic procedures is advanced maternal age, although if the father is over 55, that, too, is a strong reason for testing. A woman of 35 may object to being characterized as of advanced age, but that is what she is in relation to childbearing. Her 35-year-old eggs have been there for a long time, and their ability to divide properly into haploid, or single, cells of 23 chromosomes that can unite with the sperm's 23 chromosomes may be compromised. If the resulting diploid cell does not divide properly, that gives rise to chromosomal anomalies.

MATERNAL ALPHA-FETOPROTEIN

During the fourth week of gestation, a ridge of tissue forms in the fetus that will house the spinal cord and brain. If this ridge does not close to form a tube, called the neural tube, by day 28, a birth defect known as spina bifida results. (The imperfect closure of the spinal column means that some of the nervous system is exposed, often resulting in hydrocephalus, paralysis, and other abnormalities.) In the presence of a neural tube defect, a substance termed alpha-fetoprotein (AFP), made in the fetal brain, leaks out into the mother's circulation. Maternal blood drawn between weeks 14 to 17 of the pregnancy is tested for the presence of AFP. If the blood level is high, the fetus may have a neural tube defect, that is, spina bifida. It is also a concern if the level is low, since such a finding has been associated with Down syndrome.

It is standard screening procedure for every pregnant woman to have a blood test for maternal serum AFP, unless she is 35 or older and will later be having amniocentesis. In younger women, if the maternal serum AFP level is normal, no further testing by means of amniocentesis need be undertaken. If the test reveals decreased levels of AFP, however, amniocentesis is recommended since no one is immune to giving birth to a baby with Down syndrome; indeed, 80 percent of babies with Down syndrome are born to mothers under 35 because they do not routinely undergo prenatal genetic testing. The statistics are these: When the mother is between 15 and 19 years old, there is a one in 1,250 chance of her having a baby with Down syndrome; between 25 and 29, the likelihood is one in 1,100; at 30 it is one in 900; at 40, one in 100; at 45, one in 25.

If the maternal serum AFP is elevated, suggesting an open neural tube defect, further testing with ultrasound and amniocentesis must be done. (Ultrasound testing alone is not sufficient.) If the results of these tests are normal, it is presumed that the serum from the mother gave a false picture. We do know, however, that as the pregnancy progresses to its later stages, there is increased mortality among babies whose mothers earlier showed a high maternal serum AFP level. Thus, because of the possibility of a poor outcome, the fetus needs to be closely monitored in the later stages of pregnancy. If we fail to determine the maternal serum AFP level, we lose the marker that would have told us to keep a watchful eye on this baby until it is born.

A more comprehensive test than determination of the AFP level alone is called a "triple screen" and includes measurement of the levels of hCG (pregnancy hormone) and estrogen in the mother's blood. If the AFP level is low and the hCG level is high, this finding is suggestive of Down syndrome in the fetus. If all three are very low, the risk that the fetus has trisomy 18, another debilitating birth defect, is higher than normal.

ULTRASOUND

Ultrasound, sonogram, and *sonography* are synonyms for a test that uses sound waves, not X-rays, to produce an image—in this case, an image of the fetus inside the womb. Ultrasound can be used safely throughout pregnancy to determine the age and physical condition of the fetus.

The question of whether all pregnant women should have ultrasound testing is answered differently in Europe than it is in the United States. The European way is to schedule ultrasound testing three times (once in each trimester) in the course of a pregnancy, while in this country the National Institutes of Health (NIH), on the basis of the findings of a consensus panel, has stated that ultrasound testing during pregnancy is not necessary at all. I take issue with that, just as I take issue at the other end of the spectrum with women who wish to have several ultrasounds in order to paste the pictures in their baby book.

When ultrasound is utilized at 18 to 20 weeks, the fetal structures are large enough and defined enough for gross abnormalities to be detected. The sonographer looks to see that the skull is present in order to establish that it is not an anencephalic fetus and checks the spinal column to verify that closure has taken place and the baby will not suffer from spina bifida. The presence of such organs as the bladder, liver, and kidneys is verified, as well as the four chambers of the heart.

It should be noted that ultrasound testing has its limitations. A patient may complain, "I had an ultrasound at 16 weeks. How did they miss my baby's heart defect?" They missed it because the heart at 16 weeks is the size of a pea and there are four chambers inside it. Also, if the mother has gained a great deal of weight or is obese, sonography is not as accurate. If there is a defect in one of the chambers, usually it will be discovered, but occasionally, understandably, it is not seen.

AMNIOCENTESIS

A baby in utero is like a little frog; it lives in fluid. Cells from the baby's skin are shed into the fluid, the baby urinates into it, and the products of its metabolism go into it. Thus, the amniotic fluid is representative of the baby, and it is this fluid that is tested in amniocentesis.

Amniocentesis is carried out between 16 and 18 weeks of pregnancy. By means of ultrasound, pockets of amniotic fluid are identified, and a needle is introduced by the obstetrician through the mother's abdomen, puncturing the amniotic sac. About an ounce, 20 to 30 cc., of clear, slightly yellowish or amber fluid is withdrawn. That specimen is spun down immediately, and the cells are cultured and subjected to DNA and chromosomal analysis. Occasionally it happens that the cells do not grow and the procedure has to be repeated, but that is rare.

In addition to chromosomal analysis, a little bit of the amniotic fluid is analyzed for AFP. The level of this protein, which has earlier been determined in the mother, now is determined in the amniotic fluid. The level is high early in pregnancy but then goes down toward midpregnancy. As stated previously, if it is very low, it is an indicator for Down syndrome (the low level, some believe, is due to an underdeveloped liver caused by the extra chromosome in Down syndrome). If the level is sky-high, it is a red flag signaling the possibility of structural or chromosomal defects in the baby. Structural defects can be anencephaly or spina bifida; or an anomaly such as omphalocele, a defect in the umbilical cord; or gastroschisis, a defect in the abdominal wall that allows some of the liver and spleen and intestines to float free in the amniotic sac. To confirm the findings of the AFP test, a second test is done to determine the level of acetylcholinesterase. This test is the gold standard; it gives more trustworthy results than the test for AFP.

Patients who are leery of needles tend to ask hopefully whether ultrasound cannot give the same information as amniocentesis. The answer to that depends on which camp you are in. The ultrasonographers are inclined to say that if the ultrasound is negative, if they do not see any neural tube defect and the brain is okay, an amniocentensis is not needed. Obstetricians, on the other hand, say that the ultrasonographer is looking at a static picture that simply reveals structure; it does not give any information about the chromosomes. If there has been a clinical finding of high maternal serum AFP, an amniocentesis is imperative to identify whether there is an abnormal chromosomal makeup.

A normal complement of chromosomes for human beings is 46, or 23 pairs. In chromosomal pair 21, if there is an extra chromosome in addition to the pair, it is called trisomy 21 (*tri* for "three," *-somy* for "chromosome"); if there is an extra with pair 18, this is trisomy 18. With trisomy 18, infants rarely live longer than a year. With trisomy 21 the extra chromosome gives rise to Down syndrome. As a biology student, I thought at first that the extra chromosome would confer superior intelligence or larger stature on its possessor. Unfortunately, it is just the opposite; the extra chromosome results in mental retardation and multiple physical handicaps.

CHORIONIC VILLUS SAMPLING

Chorionic villus sampling (CVS) is the best-kept secret in obstetrics, which is a pity because it provides the earliest opportunity for prenatal diagnosis. In contrast to ultrasound and amniocentesis at 16 to 20 weeks, CVS is done in the tenth to the twelfth week of pregnancy, with the tenth week calculated as starting at nine weeks and one day.

Chorionic villi are the beginnings of the placenta. Rapidly growing, fingerlike projections in the side walls of the uterus, they look like sea kelp. By means of a soft catheter introduced vaginally and guided by ultrasound, a sample of these villi can be aspirated and sent to the laboratory for culturing. The cells are dividing very rapidly at this early stage and they grow quickly in the culture, giving results in seven days, in contrast to amniocentesis, which takes two weeks for results. As well as providing material for a chromosomal analysis, CVS allows us to rule out Tay-Sachs, sickle-cell anemia, and any inborn error of metabolism or enzymatic problem. The only thing this test does not do is establish the AFP level, but because every woman not having amniocentesis is screened with a blood test for AFP, this is not a problem.

Chorionic villus sampling yields the same information as an amniocentesis done five, six, or seven weeks later. The presence of anomalies can be confirmed at ten weeks—before the pregnancy is showing, before the woman is feeling fetal movement, and before there is the degree of bonding with the baby that is likely to have taken place by 20 weeks. Thus, if the findings give rise to a decision not to continue with the pregnancy, it can be interrupted with a

D and C with far less morbidity and psychological stress than is occasioned by a second trimester termination.

Women who are 35 or older are particularly apt candidates for CVS because of the increased incidence of fetal abnormalities in this age group. Other candidates for CVS are those who have had a previous child with Down syndrome or parents who both have a trait for Tay-Sachs disease, sickle-cell anemia, or thalassemia.

Unfortunately, most patients do not know about CVS and they may not be offered it by their obstetrician, either because he or she, too, does not know about it or has not the special training to do it or has an idea that it may cause birth defects. Some years ago, instances of limb reduction—shortened fingers or toes—began to turn up following CVS, primarily in one study in England. Those of us who are well trained in the procedure were baffled because this did not occur in our patients, but we soon realized that the problem was center-specific. Physicians at some centers either did the procedure with a non-FDA-approved catheter that was too large or did it too early in the pregnancy or had had insufficient experience with the procedure. Those of us who were experienced, used the FDA-approved catheter, and did the test at the proper time saw no increase. Consequently, we tried to say, "Well, if you did it the right way . . ." But after that seed of mistrust of a procedure is planted, it is very difficult to eradicate it. Obstetricians are still telling their patients, "You don't want CVS. The kid'll have nubbins. Let's wait for your amnio."

So the woman waits for amniocentesis, and let's say that unfortunately the test reveals trisomy 21; she has three children already and she does not want to continue with the pregnancy. But ending a pregnancy that is in the second trimester is not a simple matter of a D and C, as most people assume. Instead, the patient must go through labor and deliver the baby. Another amniocentesis can be done to instill saline into the amniotic sac to initiate labor, but the more common practice is the use of vaginal suppositories of prostaglandin to start contractions. Hopefully, labor will not last more than 24 hours until the cervix is fully dilated and the fetus is extruded, but the woman is in pain for those 24 hours.

After the uterus is emptied of the fetus, which is usually previable (not alive), the cord is cut and the fetus is sent to the pathology laboratory to confirm the presence of abnormal chromosomes. But the ordeal is not over for the mother because the placenta is still in the uterus. In a full-term pregnancy, the placenta is fully developed, and after the baby is born, it cleaves off; that is, it separates from the wall of the uterus and is delivered. But in a preterm pregnancy, often the placenta lacks the ability to separate and is stuck on the wall, making it what is called an adherent or retained placenta. The obstetrician stands by, waiting for an hour, two hours, three hours. If the placenta is still retained, the patient has to be taken to the operating room for a completion D and C. This procedure carries with it not only the risk of hemorrhage but the risk of perforating the uterus with instruments as the obstetrician struggles to separate the placenta from the wall.

RISK FACTORS IN CVS VERSUS AMNIOCENTESIS

The two main possible complications of amniocentesis are infection and leakage of the amniotic fluid. If the puncture made by the needle as it goes into the amniotic sac does not close up when the needle is withdrawn, the amniotic fluid may leak out until there is no fluid left for the baby to exist in; the baby fails to grow and the pregnancy may have to be terminated. The other possible scenario is that bacteria enter through the puncture made by the needle, infection sets in, and again the pregnancy has to be terminated.

The possible complication with CVS comes from the fact that the uterus is being entered with a catheter. The catheter is about the size of number 8 spaghetti and is very pliable, but there is the possibility that it can interfere with the fetus. When bleeding follows the procedure, the concern is whether the bleeding is coming from the placenta's having been disrupted from its little pad or whether fetal loss is about to occur. Unless a perineal pad, such as a Kotex, is soaked with bright red blood in as short a time as an hour, the bleeding is not a cause for concern. It can be compared to the bleeding that follows dental surgery: The dentist puts the gauze in and the patient takes it out when she gets home.

Some years ago there was a risk of infection with CVS, but we discovered that it came from using the same catheter more than once. If the cytogeneticist says, "Okay, you got the villi, but it's not enough material," and we have to go in again, now we know to use a fresh catheter, and the rate of infection is no higher than for amniocentesis.

Both CVS and amniocentesis, then, are *invasive procedures*, and with an invasive procedure, there is always some risk. But it is difficult to make a comparison of the risks involved for these two because there are accurate statistics for CVS but few or none for amniocentesis. There is a central registry at Jefferson Medical College in Philadelphia to which CVS tests and their outcome are reported, but comparable records are not kept for amniocentesis. The best guess seems to be that the fetal loss rate for amniocentesis is 0.6 percent and for CVS 0.8 percent—in other words, both are less than 1 percent. It is important for patients to know this in case their request for CVS testing early in pregnancy is passed off by their doctor with, "No, we'll just wait for amniocentesis; it's safer."

Such a slight difference of 0.6 as compared to 0.8 percent is interesting in view of the fact that CVS is performed early in pregnancy when the *spontaneous* rate of loss is as high as 32 percent in all pregnancies, recognized or unrecognized, and 20 percent in pregnancies confirmed by a positive pregnancy test. A third to a fifth of all pregnancies do not make it past the first weeks in any event. This is in comparison to the time period in which amniocentesis is done when the spontaneous loss rate is only one percent. Thus, to compare CVS and amniocentesis is to compare apples and oranges. Nevertheless, if amniocentesis done against a background of one percent loss has a record of 0.6 percent miscarriage, and CVS done against a background of 20 to 30 percent loss has a record of 0.8, there would seem to be little to choose between them as far as risk to the fetus is concerned and the decision should be based on other factors. My concern is that women too often cannot make the choice because they simply do not know that an alternative to amniocentesis exists, or if they hear about it, they are already 12 weeks into the pregnancy and it is too late for CVS.

Women who know about it tend to be older women of 39 or 43 who have done their homework, so I was surprised one day when a woman of 28 came, referred by a doctor who had never before sent a patient to me for CVS. I asked her how she knew about it, and she said, "My first pregnancy was a Down syndrome fetus and I went through a second trimester termination. It was absolute hell. I didn't feel I could stand to go through that again, so I asked Dr. X, who delivered me then, if there wasn't some way of finding out sooner if this baby has chromosomal problems too. He said, 'Oh, yeah, there's CVS.' I guess he didn't offer it to me sooner because it's brand new, eh?"

"It's been around since 1968," I told her.

"What! Why didn't he tell me the first time?"

I hate to think there was an economic motive, that because a lot of doctors do not know how to do CVS—which requires a maternal-fetal medicine fellowship to learn—and they do know how to do amniocentesis, the choice is not offered. But just in case, I want to get the word out as widely as possible because it is cruel to put a woman through a second trimester termination when CVS allows her to terminate, if she wishes, with a simple D and C. (A patient will sometimes ask whether, if the chromosomes are normal at 12 weeks, they will still be normal at 20 weeks. The answer is yes; the genetic makeup of the baby does not change.)

Some doctors, instead of referring a patient for CVS, will instead say to her, "Well, we'll do an early amniocentesis. We'll do it at 14 weeks instead of 16 weeks." The woman says okay. But the amount of amniotic fluid is much smaller at 14 weeks than at 16 to 18 weeks; a needle is still being introduced; and it still takes two weeks to get the results, which means that the pregnancy is then at 16 weeks and well past the time when a D and C is possible. It sounds good, but at anything more than 13 weeks, the window of opportunity for a D and C is closed. In fact, when a woman comes at 11 weeks for CVS, we ask to get the results back really fast, so that she will be no more than 12 weeks along if it happens that she arrives at a decision to terminate. Another factor against early amniocentesis is that it has been associated with a higher fetal loss rate (2.5 times higher than when done later in pregnancy) as well as orthopedic problems in the child (clubfoot).

I regret to say that some women come for CVS for gender selection, which I consider immoral. When I was new at CVS, I would see on the mother's obstetrical history "female, female, female," and I'd say, "Oh, you have three little girls, isn't that great." She'd answer, "Yeah, well, this one had better be a boy." If the CVS showed it was a boy, fine, but if it was a girl, after awhile I would get a call from the genetic counselor that Mrs. So-and-so had miscarried. Mrs. So-and-so would say, "Oh, I was lifting the groceries" or

"I fell down the porch steps," but I soon caught on to the fact that the "miscarriage" happened only when it was a girl, not when it was a boy.

GENETIC COUNSELING

If there is a family history of genetic problems, a geneticist can counsel prospective parents about the odds of their baby being affected by, for instance, mental retardation. If you go to your family reunion and little JoJo over there has a strange appearance, he may have a chromosomal problem that you would just as soon your child did not inherit, in which case you can talk to a geneticist. He or she will trace the family tree on both sides and track the transmission of the genetic defect to determine whether it is close, like first cousins, or distant, like third cousins, and whether it is likely that your child will be affected or only a remote possibility.

THE TERMINATION DECISION

With prenatal testing, we can identify both structural abnormalities and potential defects due to an extra chromosome, a missing chromosome, or a broken chromosome. For instance, a deletion of the short arm of the fifth chromosome is linked with the *cri-du-chat*, or cat cry, syndrome; along with a lot of other problems, the baby sounds like a little cat when it cries. While not knowing exactly what causes such chromosomal defects, we can detect their presence and inform the parents, who can then decide whether to continue the pregnancy.

A certain number of patients refuse testing, saying, "We're not having ultrasound or amniocentesis, Dr. Thornton, because even if something turns up, we're not going to end the pregnancy; it's against our religion." Or an older woman will say, "It's taken me so long to get pregnant that I'll take it whatever it is and just hope for the best." But if I were to accept their reasons and make no effort to persuade patients differently, I would feel I was doing them a disservice.

Instead I answer: "Whatever you choose to do is your decision, yours alone, and I would in no way attempt to intervene in it, but I do believe it is better to act from a position of knowledge than ignorance. Say that the baby has Down syndrome or spina bifida or a heart anomaly, and you decide to continue with the pregnancy. Knowing what to expect, we can have ancillary support staff present when the baby is born; it won't take us by surprise, and the baby will receive whatever special care it may need immediately."

When it is put this way, when the couple see prenatal testing simply as a source of information they can act on in the way they think best, most couples decide in favor of the testing. If the fetus does prove to have some abnormality, 7 out of 100 couples will say "Thank you, we'll take it, whatever it is," while 93 out of 100 will say "Thank you for letting us know. We're going to terminate the pregnancy tomorrow." Obstetricians do not encourage termination; we are not advocates for abortion. However, most of us feel that families should know what is coming down the pike if we have the technology to inform them of it.

This is particularly important if a couple has other children. It is one thing if the parents believe that, for themselves, the honest and noble course is to accept what fate brings, but it can be quite another for them to impose the necessity to be noble on their other children without their consent. A physically or mentally handicapped child takes time and resources away from the other family members. The parents have necessarily to be far more involved with the affected child, and this can be alienating to the normal children. At the very least, the children should be told that, "Little Johnny is going to be born with this or that. What do you think about it?" They cannot be asked to make a decision, but the family as a whole should be involved in discussing the situation because it is the family as a whole that is going to be affected, perhaps in severe, difficult, and exhausting ways.

A child with Down syndrome, for example, lacks the ability to retrieve information. Both long-term and short-term memory are basically absent, and the condition worsens with age. The child who may be a high-level retardate at 12 will show much more severe evidence of retardation by the age of 20. He or she will need lifetime care; the drain on family finances will be acute; and the parents will have to make provision in their wills to have care continued after their deaths so that the handicapped person is not consigned to an institution.

I have had women of 25 seek genetic counseling, and when I ask why, they say, "Because I don't want ever, *ever*, to deliver a child that is not normal. My parents did and it virtually destroyed the family. All their time and attention went to my affected brother, excluding the rest of us and leaving us to fend for ourselves." That is why, when an early test gives an abnormal result but the couple refuses further testing because "we are not going to abort," I do not simply accept that, as some of my colleagues do. I talk to the couple at length to ensure that they are looking at the problem in the perspective of a lifetime.

The decision whether to continue a pregnancy cannot be long delayed because hospitals around the country rarely countenance termination after 20 or 21 weeks. According to *Roe v. Wade*, termination is allowable up to 28 weeks, the time of viability, but rarely, as mentioned before, is it the policy of hospitals to permit termination after 21 weeks, unless the abnormality is incompatible with life—for example, an anencephalic fetus at 23 weeks. If the child has an anomaly compatible with life, such as hydronephrosis (enlarged kidneys), then the pregnancy must go on.

With the laboratory studies that are done between 14 and 17 weeks, with ultrasound examination, and with amniocentesis between 16 and 20 weeks, people have enough time to make up their minds unless they become bogged down in procrastination and denial. It is a different story when the pregnant woman says to herself, "I've had three kids already so I won't bother with prenatal visits with this one. I'll just wait until I have labor pains, then I'll go to the hospital." If that fourth baby is not healthy, no one knows that until it is born.

There are also patients who show up in the emergency room because they are having some bleeding, and when you ask how recently they have seen a doctor, they say this is their first visit. If they are at 26 weeks and the child has a cardiac defect or hydrocephalus, it is too bad but that is it. At 26 weeks there is nothing to be done except wait for delivery.

Having given the bad news, let me now give the good news: Only 3 to 5 percent of infants are born with major birth defects. This means that 95 to 97 percent of babies are normal and healthy. Pretty good odds, don't you think?

POINTS TO REMEMBER

- Any prospective parent can request prenatal testing. A mother 35 or older and/or a father over 55 should not fail to do so.
- The maternal serum AFP level is determined in pregnant women between weeks 14 and 17. A high level is suggestive of a neural tube defect; a low level, of Down syndrome.
- Ultrasound testing to determine the age and physical condition of the fetus is safe at any stage of pregnancy but is usually done at 18 to 20 weeks.
- Amniocentesis, carried out between 16 and 18 weeks, involves withdrawal of amniotic fluid by means of a needle inserted through the mother's abdomen. The fluid undergoes DNA and chromosomal analysis.
- A CVS procedure, done between weeks 10 and 12, provides the earliest opportunity for prenatal diagnosis. Fetal abnormalities can be detected while the pregnancy can still be terminated with a simple D and C.
- Termination of pregnancy, if decided on after amniocentesis in the second trimester, necessitates labor and delivery and carries the risk of a retained placenta.
- The risk of loss of the fetus is less than 1 percent for both CVS and amniocentesis.
- To forgo prenatal testing because the parents intend to accept whatever fate has in store means that preparations cannot be made in the event the baby requires special care.
- The impact of a defective child on family life and the other children in the family, both immediate and long-term, should be carefully weighed before a decision for or against termination of the pregnancy is made.

9

MEDICAL CONDITIONS IN PREGNANCY

❧

HIV • SURGICAL CONDITIONS • MALIGNANCY • DIA-
BETES • AUTO-IMMUNE DISEASE • Rh-NEGATIVE •

Women will spend days or weeks looking into buying a house or car
but enter into pregnancy without giving it much advance thought.
Obviously, the wiser course would be to do a bit of planning before
you stop taking the Pill or using the diaphragm. You can make certain your nutrition is optimal so the fetus can get what it needs from
the body's store of nutrients—although, actually, the baby is prepro-
grammed to take what it needs and it is you who will develop the
anemia or, in later years, the osteoporosis if you are not well nour-
ished. Because a possible cause of miscarriage is infection, it is a good
idea to have cultures done to check for the presence of group B beta
streptococcus or *Mycoplasma, Ureaplasma,* and *chlamydia*; such infections can and should be treated before you become pregnant.
Depending on your heritage, you and your husband can be checked
to determine if you are carriers for Tay-Sachs, sickle-cell anemia, or
thalassemia.

It is also sensible to have a preconceptual evaluation in which
your blood type is determined; you are screened for toxoplasmosis if
you have cats or eat steak tartare or drink goat's milk; and you are
tested for antibodies to rubella (German measles), rubeola (regular
measles), and varicella (chickenpox). You do not want to be six
weeks' pregnant, kiss a young nephew, come down with German
measles, and have to terminate a pregnancy that might otherwise
have gone along just fine. Vaccination protects against these diseases, but it must be done when you are not pregnant, not after you
become pregnant, because the vaccine contains live viruses that may
possibly damage the fetus.

Any virus and any bacteria can potentially cross over the placenta. The placenta is nice and plush and lush—it is very, very vascular—and whatever the mother is infected with usually finds it a fertile ground to multiply in. Thus the infection gets to the fetus, whether it is syphilis, Lyme disease, chlamydia, toxoplasmosis, or any of a number of other infections, including HIV.

HIV

The Center for Disease Control reports, "HIV (human immunodeficiency virus) infection has become a leading cause of morbidity and mortality among women, the population accounting for the most rapid increase in cases of acquired immune deficiency syndrome (AIDS) in recent years." This means that HIV has also become a leading cause of death for young children because of mother-to-infant transmission.

Many of the babies born to women with HIV die, but not all. The baby who tests positive at birth may test negative in a year because the baby, although the virus has crossed the placenta, has not contracted the disease. Thus, babies are tested at regular intervals to see whether they are truly infected or whether the first test was a reflection of the mother's positive infectivity.

The risk of transmission of HIV from mother to baby is greatly reduced if the mother is treated with zidovudine, more commonly known as AZT. The greatest benefit from AZT comes if the mother's positive status is diagnosed either before she becomes pregnant or early in the pregnancy. Unfortunately, a woman cannot be tested for HIV without her consent, so the fact that she is infected may be unknown and treatment to protect the fetus is not started.

SURGICAL CONDITIONS

It used to be said—and written in medical textbooks—that pregnant women were at increased risk of death from appendicitis or a gallbladder attack. Now we know the reason for the increased risk: They were not treated like ordinary people. Physicians believed that because a woman was pregnant, they could not operate on her, and whatever the disease was, it often kept advancing until it killed her. Now when a physician consults an obstetrician about a pregnant patient, the answer he or she gets is, "Do what you would normally do if she weren't pregnant." It may be a little tricky to remove a gallbladder or appendix, but the surgeon can move the uterus aside and do what needs to be done. If the pregnancy is advanced, medications are often given prophylactically to prevent or stop contractions, but otherwise, if the mother is well oxygenated during the surgery, there are seldom any problems.

MALIGNANCY

Whether cancer in a pregnant woman should be treated in the same fashion as in a nonpregnant woman depends somewhat on when the malignancy is discovered. From the start of pregnancy through the twelfth week, the organs of the baby are being formed: the limbs, the brain, the liver, et cetera. If within that time the cancer treatment calls for the mother to be given high doses of chemotherapy or to be exposed to extremely high doses of radiation, the organs of the growing fetus are likely to be malformed and will remain malformed throughout the pregnancy. So one would prefer not to treat a cancer patient until after the twelfth week. But if the mother is going to die without the treatment, there is little point in protecting the fetus.

When I was at The New York Hospital, pregnant patients at Sloan-Kettering with brain cancer who were being treated with anti-cancer agents would ask me as the perinatologist, "How is the baby?" I would say, in effect, "If you are not on medication, you have little chance for survival, so we have to give you the drugs and just keep our fingers crossed that they won't affect the baby."

Often there would be a whole team of physicians for one woman and we would pull her through, and she and the baby—thank God— would both be okay. Then she would come back and say she intended to have another baby. We doctors would look at each other, thinking, "Is she crazy? Does she have any idea how close she was to dying?" Denial, refusal to face reality, can be very strong.

I recently did a D and C on a patient who was 11 weeks pregnant. She kept being nauseated and was vomiting and so dizzy that she could not keep her balance, and no drug was helping. It was assumed this was due to hyperemesis gravidarum (see chapter 5), but someone suggested doing an MRI just to be sure, and there it was: a cerebellar tumor in the brain. So, the patient is 11 weeks pregnant and has a just-discovered brain tumor; how should she be treated? The perinatologists asked the oncologists what they would do if she were not pregnant. Chemotherapy, they said. Then that is what you must do, we told them, even if you cannot wait until 12 weeks, because there is no use worrying about the fetus if the mother is not going to make it. A surgeon offered, "We can go in and do neurosurgery to see exactly the extent and type of tumor, whether it is benign or malignant, in order to best direct chemotherapy if it is malignant or possibly remove it if it is benign." We answered, "Surgery, believe it or not, would be the better option—much better than giving medication that crosses over the placenta."

Immediately before the surgery, the baby was scanned with ultrasound and there was no fetal heart; the baby had died. The timing of chemotherapy was now a moot point because, for whatever reason, the baby was gone. Had the baby been viable, we would have asked the oncologists to wait after the operation until the twelfth week before instituting chemotherapy.

A baby beyond the first trimester is rugged, really resistant to damage. In the old days, we were reluctant to treat the pregnant woman for fear of harming her fetus, and often as a consequence she died. Now we are getting bolder, and not only is the mother living but so is the baby. Particularly after 20 weeks' gestation, if it is not going to kill the mother, it is not going to kill the baby or even damage it. The fetus has a liver, just as the mother does, and the fetus usually has the necessary enzymes to break the chemicals down, just as the mother has, with the exception of alcohol dehydrogenase. (As described previously, in unborn babies there is no enzyme to metabolize alcohol, and the alcohol can linger in the baby's body, especially in the brain, to cause fetal alcohol syndrome.)

DIABETES

Diabetes in pregnancy, known as gestational diabetes, is not uncommon and is different from the diabetes seen in nonpregnant adults or even in juveniles, since in pregnancy it develops by a different mechanism. However, the result is the same in that the pancreas, the organ that produces insulin, cannot keep up with the demands of the body and consequently there are high levels of glucose (sugar) in the blood.

During pregnancy, because glucose is essential to the baby's growth and development, the need of the fetus for glucose is paramount. Ordinarily, excess glucose is stored in a person's liver and peripherally as fat through the action of insulin, but in pregnancy the placenta produces "anti-insulin" hormones to make sure that whatever excess glucose the mother has is not stored in her tissues but is instead directed through the placenta for the fetus to make use of. The fetus, acting as a sugar "sink," craves glucose and the placenta obliges.

As the pregnancy advances, the placenta becomes larger; in so doing, it produces more and more anti-insulin hormones to block the storage function of insulin. The more the placenta secretes anti-insulin hormones, the more the mother's pancreas counters with increasing levels of insulin. It is rather like a tug-of-war over who will get the glucose, the mother or the baby. In gestational diabetes, the mother's pancreas simply becomes exhausted, and any excess glucose in her body is not stored but is allowed to circulate unchecked. Under normal circumstances, the kidneys do not permit glucose to escape from the body through the urine, but if the amount of glucose becomes elevated beyond a certain point, the excretion of glucose cannot be prevented and the pregnant woman starts "spilling" sugar in her urine.

Initial treatment usually involves reducing the amount of carbohydrates eaten by the mother. The patient may be referred to a nutritionist for counseling, and an American Diabetic Association diet is prescribed, with the number of calories to be consumed calculated on the basis of her weight. A change in the mother's diet is often all that is needed, but if after several days her blood sugar level is still elevated, injections of insulin are prescribed because overly high levels of glucose are not good for the baby.

The baby may become huge in utero if the excess levels of glucose are allowed to continue. When there are high circulating levels of glucose, the baby's pancreas also produces insulin, and this insulin triggers the production of fat cells in the baby. The more glucose in the mother, the more glucose in the baby. Infants of diabetic mothers are chubby, weighing 10 or 11 pounds. While they may look like cherubs, these babies have numerous life-threatening problems in the nursery, and there is a greatly increased incidence of still-birth among the infants of diabetic mothers.

Mothers are anxious to know whether they will still be diabetic and have to use insulin after the baby is born. Thankfully, in the overwhelming majority of patients the answer is no. The placenta is delivered along with the baby, and the mother's pancreas can return to normal functioning because it is no longer being challenged by the anti-insulin hormone elaborated by the placenta. Obesity in the mother, however, may tilt the scales toward a persistence of the high blood levels of glucose, and thus diabetes.

AUTO-IMMUNE DISEASE

An auto-immune disease, like lupus, while it does not attack the fetus directly, does attack the placenta, causing the blood vessels to become clogged, which means that there is a poor support mechanism for the fetus. A mother with lupus is placed on a regimen of baby aspirin throughout her pregnancy to lessen or prevent the little blood clots that plug the vessels in the placenta. Minimal amounts of heparin, an anticlotting agent, may also be prescribed to prevent an early pregnancy loss or later stillbirth. Interestingly enough, sometimes the first sign of a mother's having an auto-immune disorder is a heart irregularity discovered in the baby, either in the doctor's office or by means of ultrasound.

RH-NEGATIVE

Rh factor, so called because it was first found in the blood of Rhesus monkeys, is defined as any one of a group of inheritable antigens in the red blood cells of most persons, who are then said to be Rh-positive. By the same token, someone who lacks the antigens is said to be Rh-negative. Seventy percent of Rh-negative mothers are married to Rh-positive men. When a mother is Rh-negative and the father Rh-positive, the baby is most likely to be Rh-positive. In a first pregnancy, this usually is not a problem because the baby goes undetected by the mother's immune system. However, at the time of delivery a large amount of the baby's blood can become admixed with the mother's blood via the delivery of the placenta. For the first time the two different Rh factors meet, and the mother's blood does not recognize the Rh-positive cells. Belatedly—the baby is already born—the mother's immune system reacts to the incompatible blood, and its defense mechanism is activated. "It's an alien! How did we let that different cell slip through? This will never happen again! We're going to mount an attack against anybody else who is Rh-positive and dares to come in here." A second pregnancy occurs, the mother is still married to the Rh-positive father, and this time the Rh-positive baby provokes the antibody response of the mother's immune system.

The antibodies march across the placenta like soldiers and destroy the red blood cells of the growing fetus. The baby becomes profoundly anemic and starts trying to compensate for this anemia by making more red blood cells in its own little bone marrow and liver and spleen. These immature red blood cells are called erythroblasts, and erythroblastosis fetalis is the medical term for what are known as "blue babies."

Professors of mine at Columbia were the discoverers of RhoGAM, which revolutionized the practice of obstetrics in the 1960s by insuring against the birth of blue babies. Working with male prisoners at Sing Sing who had high levels of Rh-positive antibodies in their systems, they extracted the antibodies, sterilized and purified them, and came up with an immunoglobulin called RhoGAM. RhoGAM is a gamma globulin given to the Rh-negative mother to block recognition by her immune system of a foreign invader, that is, the Rh-positive fetus. Since RhoGAM became available, the proportion of babies born with erythroblastosis has declined to less than one percent.

In the early days of its availability, RhoGAM was given immediately after delivery, just as soon as it was determined that the mother was Rh-negative and the baby Rh-positive. It was presumed that if their blood had admixed, her reaction could only be blocked if the RhoGAM was given within three days. Thus, if an Rh-negative mother delivered and through some error it was not detected until two weeks later that the baby was Rh-positive, the thinking was "It's too late now. We can't give her the RhoGAM." But that proved to be a fallacy. A mother can be three weeks out, and if her blood is drawn and she does not yet have the antibodies, she can receive the RhoGAM injection. How did the fallacy arise? In the original study, the Sing Sing inmates were let out of prison to go to Columbia for just 72 hours, so three days became the time period in which RhoGAM was known to be effective. Finally somebody thought to test the assumption, and now we give it at any time. If a woman is known to be Rh-negative, we give it at 28 weeks of gestation and again at delivery. If she has an invasive procedure, like CVS or amniocentesis, in which there is a possibility of an admixture of mother's and baby's blood, it is also given then.

POINTS TO REMEMBER

- A medical evaluation prior to pregnancy is recommended to prevent later problems.
- An HIV-positive woman should be treated with AZT during pregnancy to reduce the risk of transmitting the virus to the baby.
- Surgery during pregnancy for such conditions as appendicitis or gallbladder disease presents little risk.
- When malignancy is present in the pregnant woman, it is preferable, but not always possible, to postpone treatment until after the first trimester when the baby's organs are being formed.
- Uncontrolled gestational diabetes can cause stillbirth.
- Gestational diabetes can usually be controlled by diet and will disappear after the birth of the baby.
- Auto-immune disease can cause prematurity or stillbirth by affecting the placenta.
- When the mother is Rh-negative and the father is Rh-positive, treatment of the mother with RhoGAM prevents the birth of a "blue baby."

10

WHERE'S MY EPIDURAL?

ॐ

WHATEVER HAPPENED TO LAMAZE? • THE TRAINING •
THE DISILLUSIONMENT • EPIDURAL ANESTHESIA • THE
RISKS • THE TIMING • FOLEY BAGS • "I HAVE A LITTLE
LIST" • NO IV, PLEASE • NO ENEMA, PLEASE • NO EPI-
SIOTOMY, PLEASE • TEARING UP THE LIST •

In the 1950s, "twilight sleep" to ease the pain of childbirth was in
vogue. Then came the 60s, and a backlash against anesthesia set in.
"We want to be there, we want to experience labor," women said.
"You doctors are not going to have control over us. We don't want
to have drugs in our bodies." At this juncture the Lamaze technique
of natural childbirth became popular.

WHATEVER HAPPENED TO LAMAZE?

The Training. The Lamaze training is described in a little book
called *Six Practical Lessons to an Easier Childbirth*, by Elisabeth Bing. My
obstetrician sent me to Mrs. Bing when I was having my children in
the 1970s, and I can still quote what Mrs. Bing said then: "The question is not whether you're going to have pain—you are. The question
is how you're going to deal with it. A contraction is like a big wave
coming. You can't stop the wave, so are you going to tense up and be
battered by it, really smacked by it, or are you going to ride it?"

The way to ride it, Mrs. Bing taught, is to focus on something
outside yourself while breathing deeply and counting these deep
breaths in a cadence of four—one, two, three, four—in, out, in, out.
The husband, who also attends the Lamaze classes, is instructed to
squeeze his wife's knee to simulate the pain of a contraction while

the wife tries to focus her attention elsewhere. Shearwood, my husband, is an orthopedic surgeon and has a hand as big as a mitt and as strong as a vise. When he squeezed my knee, I thought I was going to die. "This is silly. This is awful. This is useless," he kept muttering, until one night we were practicing at home and he started squeezing mildly, then harder, then harder. I was focusing on a light switch across the room. "Why aren't you hollering?" Shearwood demanded. "Honey," I answered calmly, "you can squeeze all night as far as I'm concerned." That turned both our heads around. Now we knew that the Lamaze training worked.

The Disillusionment. I had both my children with only a bit of Demerol to see me through, which made me an enthusiast for the training. With many other women also having the same positive experience, the demand for Lamaze training grew, which brought more and more teachers into the field. Unfortunately, not all of them were well qualified. From what I began hearing from my patients, I learned that it was common for the training to degenerate into more of a social occasion and gossip session than a learning experience. The predictable result was patients who were not well prepared. Many women, when they came into the hospital in labor, were tense and stiff; the dilatation of the cervix did not proceed normally; and when a contraction came along, the patient could not ride out the pain.

This led to the popularity of epidural anesthesia, which was developed around this time. An epidural is the controlled delivery of anesthetic drugs via a pump system inserted in the dura, or covering, of the spine. Its advantage is that it produces not unconsciousness but numbness from the waist down. The patient is awake for the delivery of her baby, but the pain of labor is wiped out.

"This is great!" women enthused. "This is the answer." The fame of epidural anesthesia spread, and now there is scarcely a pregnant woman who comes into the obstetrician's office without saying, "I want an epidural, of course." Unfortunately, without being in the least aware of it, what they are also saying is, in effect, "After me, the baby comes first."

EPIDURAL ANESTHESIA

When I am the obstetrician and a pregnant woman announces that she wishes to have an epidural for the delivery of her child, I listen, I nod, and then I say, "There are some facts about epidural anesthesia that you should be aware of."

The Risks. The most important fact is that epidural anesthesia is not risk-free. Its widespread use has resulted in an increase in cesarean sections, in forceps deliveries, and in postdelivery bladder problems. A recent study traces 152 maternal deaths to the use of epidural anesthesia. In my own practice, I use an epidural when and if appropriate, but I caution my patients not to think of it as a harmless substitute for Lamaze training—which is still the best way to go—and not to expect its routine use.

Routine use is, unfortunately, all too common. In a typical situation, a patient in labor comes into the hospital, the cervix is only one centimeter dilated, which means the patient is in a very early stage of labor. She yells, "It hurts! It hurts!" The anesthesiologist puts the epidural in, and the anesthetic agent is started. The patient now does not feel the pain of labor and she loves it. So does the anesthesiologist because his or her fee is one hundred dollars per hour for all the time the anesthesia is running even though he or she does not stay with the patient—a nurse monitors the flow. If the patient is in labor for 23 hours, it is a very expensive procedure, although that does not count with most patients because an insurance company is paying the bill.

Far more important than the cost is the fact that the pump is delivering an anesthetic agent, a drug. That drug dripping into the patient's bloodstream crosses the placenta and reaches the baby. The agent that is numbing the nerves that exit the spinal column in the mother may have an adverse effect on the baby's heart, causing it to slow. The fetal heart that has been going bah-bah-bah-bah now begins to go bah . . . bah . . . bah . . . bah, and suddenly the obstetrician is crossing her fingers and saying to herself, "Oh, wow, I hope the rate comes back up again."

She does not know whether the slowed heart rate is due to the anesthesia or whether the cord is wrapped around the baby's neck, depriving it of oxygen. She rolls the mother on her side, and back to the other side, and up and down, to see if the baby's heart rate will come back up. She waits one minute, two minutes. Nothing happens. She cannot wait any longer; the baby may be strangling. She has to do a cesarean section. She operates. The baby comes out crying and healthy. It is fine; no cord around its neck. Everything would have been all right, a cesarean would not have been needed, if it had not been for the epidural anesthesia.

That is one of the risks. Another, this one for the mother, is that the anesthesia can go too high. The numbness is only supposed to be lumbar, below the belly button; if it goes higher it paralyzes the respiratory muscles, the woman cannot breathe, and she has to be put on a respirator. This is another piece of information that does not make the six o'clock news when people rave about epidurals.

The Timing. By now it may seem that I am totally against epidurals, but really what I am against is their being started too early in labor and continuing over many hours. If the patient is at a midpoint in labor where the cervix is dilated to 5 centimeters, the contractions are coming strongly, Demerol is not working, and the patient feels she must have an anesthetic, I go along with her. I have told her what the risks are, and if she says, "I want an epidural," it is her body and her baby.

I turn the epidural off, though, in the last stage of labor when the cervix is at ten centimeters and fully dilated because, if the anesthetic continues to flow, the patient cannot feel the contractions and does not push hard to get the baby out. A patient with the epidural still running looks at the monitor along with the nurse; the nurse says, "Contraction is coming now," the patient says "Okay," and pushes, but not strongly and very little happens. When the patient can feel the contraction, on the other hand, natural forces gives her the impetus to push. It is like having a bowel movement that you *have* to get out of your body; the patient pushes with a much stronger expulsive force and the baby is born sooner. When the mother does not have a natural incentive to push, the obstetrician may have to use forceps or a vacuum extractor to help the baby out.

From the time of full cervical dilatation until the baby is delivered averages 50 minutes for a first baby, 20 minutes for a second. But the obstetrician will wait as long as two hours for the baby to come. Then, if the mother has pushed and pushed and pushed and still has not delivered, Mother Nature is saying the baby is too big; it is not going to be born in time, before its oxygen supply gets too low, and the obstetrician has to do a cesarean section.

Doctors are sometimes criticized for this timing. People say, "The poor woman pushed and pushed for hours, and *then* they had the nerve to finally do a C-section. Why didn't they do it in the first place?" The reason is that obstetricians are trained to allow the sequence of events to unfold naturally—the word *obstetrics* comes from the Latin *ad stare*, "to stand by." Mother Nature knows what she is doing (most of the time), and only after all natural means have been exhausted does the obstetrician intervene.

Two hours is the usual cutoff point because the doctor knows that the longer the mother pushes, the poorer will be the outcome for the baby. But when an epidural is running, the doctor extends the time to three hours because the mother's expulsive efforts are so minimal that it is necessary to wait an hour longer to see if the baby will come naturally.

Foley Bags. If, after three hours, the birth is natural, the baby's head has been banging against the mother's perineum all that time, which means it is likely that the mother's bladder has been traumatized and is limp, flaccid, and does not remember what it is supposed to do. The mother should urinate within four hours after delivery; instead, she says, "I don't feel anything. I don't feel like I need to go."

A nurse catheterizes her and drains a lot of urine. Six hours go by and still the patient feels no urge. The nurse catheterizes her again and takes out a pint of fluid, an amount that will make the average person say urgently, "I have to go to the bathroom!" But the patient still does not feel anything, and the bladder, having gone over the 500 cc. mark, does not snap back; it gets bigger and bigger and bigger until the next time it may have 1000 cc. in it. So now the catheter has to be left in. It is clamped for three and a half hours to allow the urine to collect, then the clamp is released and the bladder is drained. This clamping and unclamping is continued for two or three days, and medication is given, all with the hope of persuading the bladder to remember what it is supposed to do. If it does not, the patient goes home from the hospital with a Foley bag. Eventually the bladder will right itself, but by that time the patient may believe that having an epidural was not really worth the consequences.

There are still other possible consequences. Women may experience an increase in backaches and headaches after an epidural-assisted delivery and may notice some weakness in the legs. Rare but severe complications during delivery can include a precipitous drop in blood pressure, convulsions, and respiratory or cardiac arrest.

"I HAVE A LITTLE LIST"

No IV, Please. On her initial visit to the obstetrician, the pregnant woman may bring a list of what she wants and does not want. Epidural anesthesia is usually first on the list, and after discussing the pros and cons of that, often her next statement is: "I don't want an IV in. I want to be able to walk around."

I sympathize with her feeling. But I have to point out that when labor starts, she is not likely to be eating a Blimpie or sending out for a sirloin. So it becomes a question of where she is going to get the nutrients and the fluid and glucose to see her through the hours and hours of labor.

"You're allowed to drink, aren't you?" she asks.

"Not much. Ice chips is about it because if you have anything more, you're likely to vomit and the stuff gets in your lungs."

To console her, I concede that in the early stages of labor, it does not really matter whether she has an IV in. But the picture changes in active labor when she will not be eating or drinking. Without an IV supplying fluid and glucose, she will become dehydrated and her condition will most likely begin to go downhill. But there is another, even more important reason for an intravenous line to be in place, which is that the obstetrician may need to have immediate access to a vein. Bleeding can happen very rapidly in a delivery, and when it does, veins collapse. Trying to start an IV to give fluids, blood, or medications, and being unable to get into a vein creates an emergency situation. Patient and doctor are suddenly in a huge amount of trouble (see chapter 13).

No Enema, Please. With this explanation the patient crosses "no IV" off her list and proceeds to the next item, which is usually, "I've heard about the enemas. I don't want an enema."

Again I sympathize. Nobody likes enemas. But if it is any consolation, at least it is not as bad as it was in my medical student days when enemas were given to stimulate labor and were known as the three h's: high, hot, and a heck of a lot. If a woman's labor was lagging, she would be given a hot water, hot soapsuds enema, and when she expelled it, her labor would pick up, but it was not a very pleasant experience. I used to think to myself, "Gee, I hope I never have to go through that."

The high, hot, and hellish enema is gone now, but a Fleet enema is administered to clean out the lower bowel. Without it, in the final stage of labor, when the patient is pushing and pushing, if there is fecal material in the bowel, it comes out too, and not only spills on the baby but greatly increases the risk of infection if an episiotomy is necessary.

"Oh," the woman may say at this point, "I thought it was just abusive treatment."

On the contrary, it is a sensible precaution taken to keep the field as clean as possible, which is also the reason for shaving the pubic hair—although, again, that approach has been moderated. As a student, I never did understand why the shaving had to be total, and now that has changed too. All that is shaved is the area the baby is coming through. If the patient needs to have an episiotomy, which is an incision to enlarge the vulvar opening, it is too late then to shave the area because the baby's head is right there. And after the baby is born and the incision is being sewn up, it makes things doubly difficult if hair has to be picked out from inside the suture repair line.

No Episiotomy, Please. It is little things like shaving that keep the obstetrician out of trouble and the patient from returning to the hospital later with an infected episiotomy, which is a royal mess.

An episiotomy does not have to be done—and it is not, of course—if the vagina will stretch enough for the baby to come through. But if the baby's head is larger than the opening and the obstetrician does not make an adequate cut from the vagina to the top of the rectum to release the pressure, the baby's head can pop everything. The whole area is as ripped and lacerated and bleeding as though a hand grenade has exploded, and it is a terrific job to sew everything up again. The most unpleasant result is if the levator ani muscle around the rectum has been badly torn. The mother may lose fecal continence, perhaps for months, until an effective repair of the sphincter can be attempted.

The patient who says, "I don't want an episiotomy. Don't cut me!" may be making a choice between a clean surgical cut that can be neatly repaired or a jagged rip that may not stop short of the anus and is the devil to patch up. Or she may guess correctly that the baby's head will come through without tearing tissues but the long-term consequence can be that she is rolling up her bladder when she is 50 years old because all the ligaments have been so stretched. Whether or not to have an episiotomy is really not a choice to be made in advance but a clinical decision to be made on the spot as the obstetrician sees the situation develop. (See chapter 11.)

TEARING UP THE LIST

Explaining all this, talking out concerns, correcting the misinformation that women pick up through hearsay, and, most of all, countering the suspicion that doctors do some things just to be arbitrary, takes time. I usually schedule an hour appointment with a newly pregnant woman, especially if it is her first baby. By the end of the hour, after I have explained why Lamaze training is worthwhile, why epidural anesthesia is not an automatic given, and why we obstetricians do what we do, the patient generally crumples the list of demands she arrived with and throws it in the wastebasket.

But sometimes a patient does not throw away her list, still convinced that the relationship between obstetrician and patient is necessarily adversarial rather than the deepest sort of cooperative enterprise. In such instances I suggest that the patient consult another obstetrician because I need her to trust me and know that every decision I make will be in what I honestly believe is her best interest and that of a healthy baby.

POINTS TO REMEMBER

- A "drug-free" birth by means of Lamaze training is preferable.
- Epidural anesthesia provides superior pain relief during labor.
- The disadvantages of epidural anesthesia are:
  - Anesthetic crosses the placenta, possibly causing fetal distress and emergency cesarean section.
  - Anesthesia reduces the mother's incentive to push, which may necessitate the use of forceps or vacuum extractor or a cesarean section.
  - Possible postdelivery loss of bladder function.
  - Possible postdelivery increase in backaches, headaches, and lower limb weakness.
  - More severe complications can include convulsions, respiratory or cardiac arrest, and profound drop in blood pressure.
- An IV, enema, shaving of the pubic hair, and an episiotomy are prophylactic, not punitive, measures and are designed to contribute to a trouble-free delivery.

11

IT'S NOT OVER UNTIL THE FAT BABY SINGS—LABOR AND DELIVERY

❧

THE FEMALE PELVIS • THE AMNIOTIC SAC • MATERNAL AND FETAL MONITORS • PITOCIN • LABOR • STATIONS • EPISIOTOMY • THE BABY'S FIRST BREATH • THE BABY'S ARRIVAL • BONDING • APGAR SCORES • THE OBSTETRI-CIAN AND THE NEONATALOGIST • THE THIRD STAGE OF LABOR • EPISIOTOMY REPAIR • THE FATHER IN THE DELIVERY ROOM • LDRP ROOMS • THE FOURTH STAGE • POSTPARTUM CHECKUP

Vaginal deliveries are the natural way for babies to arrive in the world. Women's bodies are programmed to reproduce, and every-thing clicks and flicks and switches and starts and stops toward the goal of a vaginal delivery. If one of the steps goes awry, then we have to think about cesarean sections and the like, but most of the time the body knows exactly what to do and does it efficiently.

THE FEMALE PELVIS

Unlike the male pelvis, which is somewhat triangular and has sharp spines, the female pelvis is framed for a vaginal delivery in that it is nice and round, with bones that are separated, ready for a little kid to shoot through. This gynecoid female pelvis is the average, but there are other types as well. Some women have a pelvis closer in shape to the male, short and stubby and angulated; this type is called an android pelvis and often occasions a cesarean delivery. There is also the flattened, or platypelloid, pelvis, which is oval, like an egg. The round head of a baby trying to get through such a pelvis is not going to make it, and the cephalopelvic (fetal head to maternal pelvis) disproportion necessitates a cesarean. Still another shape of pelvis is the anthropoid, which is often linked to ethnicity in that many black women have this type. Here, the fullness of the pelvis comes in the bottom part. Since the biggest part of the baby's head is in the back, and with the twists and turns of labor, the largest part of the head goes where there is the most space, the baby tends to arrive sunny-side up, that is, with its eyes turned toward the ceiling and the back of its head toward the floor (the more usual way is for the eyes to be facing the floor). Labor is more prolonged with this type of delivery, called occiput posterior, and can be hard on the mother because the back of the baby's head is ramming against her coccyx (tailbone). But unlike the flat pelvis and the android, the anthropoid pelvis is not likely to necessitate a cesarean section.

If the pelvis is visualized as a bowl, the goal for the baby's head is to get to the bottom of the bowl—call it the Superbowl for babies. The goal posts can be wide and hospitable to the baby, as in the gynecoid pelvis, or the pelvis can be android and make a goal line stand that conveys, "There's no way this kid's head is going to get through here." In the latter instance the mother may progress to full dilation, but then when it is time for her to push the head out of the bowl, she pushes and pushes and pushes, the baby's head bumps and bumps and bumps against the pelvic bones, two or three hours go by, but the baby cannot get born. The only way it can score is via a cesarean.

THE AMNIOTIC SAC

What is commonly referred to as the "bag of waters" is technically known as the amniotic sac, a thin membrane within the uterus that is filled with the amniotic fluid in which the baby lives. To picture it, imagine the thick, hard rubber muscle that is the uterus; inside that is a balloon filled with water, and inside that is the baby. The fluid so protects the baby that it is rare for trauma to reach the fetus. The amount of fluid in the amniotic sac increases as the pregnancy goes on until, at approximately 34 weeks, it measures about a quart. Then, after 34 weeks, the amount begins to decrease because the baby is getting larger, the placenta is getting older, and the hydrodynamics are changing. This is why we become concerned about overdue babies. For the lungs to develop properly, the fluid should be clear, but the baby is urinating and defecating inside the amniotic sac, and when the amount of fluid decreases, the fluid tends to become thick and discolored rather than remaining clear.

If the amniotic sac ruptures before term, the cause may be a bacterial infection that irritates the membranes and reduces their tensile strength. When the membranes rupture at, say, four months' gestation and the amniotic fluid is lost, the prognosis for the baby is exceedingly poor because amniotic fluid needs to be present for the lungs to develop. Furthermore, if there is no fluid, the uterus presses close to the baby and the baby cannot move around and develop its muscles. If the muscles cannot go to full extension, when the baby is delivered, it does not do well at all. If the membranes rupture at 28 weeks, we hope the baby can go to term, but in 80 percent of mothers, the time from the rupture of the membranes until delivery is seven days. Only 20 percent are lucky enough to continue on. What happens is that the uterine environment is sterile until the membranes break, but then bacteria happily travel into the new playground and start multiplying. The mother develops a fever, contractions follow, and we have to deliver the baby.

A second concern, in addition to infection, is prolapse of the cord. With rupture of the membranes, the cervix may be two or three centimeters dilated and the umbilical cord can fall through. For this reason, patients are asked to come to the hospital when their waters break. The patient's mother may say, "You're not having contractions, you're not in labor yet, so just stay home," and unfortunately some doctors agree, but the danger is that there may be an occult prolapse of the cord, that is, some part of the cord has herniated through the cervix unbeknownst to the patient and is being squeezed. Although I am sometimes accused of clucking over patients like a mother hen, I do not want my patient to call me, saying, "It's funny but I don't feel the baby moving too much anymore." I believe it is wisest to err on the side of caution and hospitalize the mother so that she can be monitored for infection and the status of the baby checked.

Normally, however, the membranes do not break until the start of labor, or until the obstetrician ruptures them deliberately, or until there is a need to thread fetal and uterine monitors into the uterus.

The obstetrician uses an Amnihook, an instrument that looks like a crochet needle and is long enough to go through the vagina and cervix, to nick the membranes and release the amniotic fluid. It is important that the fluid be examined to see whether it is clear or whether it is green or has blood in it.

What can make the amniotic fluid green is the presence of meconium, which is the excrement of the fetus. Given that the baby has been in the amniotic fluid all these many weeks and the fluid has remained clear, why should it suddenly be green? Usually it is because the baby's anal sphincter has opened up as a result of stress, making the presence of meconium a warning sign that the baby may be suffering from low oxygen levels. While we do not go immediately to a cesarean section, we do monitor the baby very carefully. Adding to the particulate matter in the amniotic fluid is a cold cream–like substance, known as vernix, that has been protecting the skin of the baby in utero and is now being sloughed off. The stressed baby is swallowing this dense amniotic fluid, and when it is born, the meconium in the trachea and in the lungs can give it severe breathing problems known as meconium aspiration syndrome.

MATERNAL AND FETAL MONITORS

In the course of labor, an external monitor in the form of a strap is put on the mother's abdomen at the top of the uterus. When the uterus contracts, the abdomen billows up, and that increase in tightness is registered on the machine. The reading tells us that the patient is having a contraction, but it does not indicate the strength of the contraction or how long it lasts, so an internal monitor is eventually necessary. The internal monitor works like a hydraulic system; every time the patient has a contraction, the contraction displaces the amniotic fluid, and that translates from centimeters of water into millimeters of mercury, giving the depth and intensity of the contraction and indicating whether, when the contraction goes down, it is returning to the baseline. The contraction, for example, starts at zero, goes up to 50, and comes back down to zero. But sometimes it comes back down only to 25 or 30. It does not return to the baseline, indicating that the uterus has a high basal tone and is not relaxing all the way. If Pitocin is being given to stimulate labor, the administration is stopped, and since Pitocin has a half-life of three minutes, meaning that its effect is gone in that amount of time, the baseline should soon return to zero. If it does not, because of the danger of amniotic fluid embolism (see chapter 13), the baby is delivered by cesarean section.

In addition to the monitor inside the uterus, a second monitor is also introduced through the vagina and attached to the baby's head to register the baby's heart rate, allowing us to pick up signs of fetal distress quickly and making intrapartum (during labor) deaths all but unknown.

PITOCIN

Pitocin is the proprietary name of synthetic oxytocin, the hormone that prompts uterine contractions. It is administered when a woman's contractions are weak or nonexistent. Pitocin-induced contractions simulate the natural pattern of contraction and relaxation of the uterus.

Before Pitocin, women would have prolonged labor for days, and babies would undergo so much stress that they would be delivered in an obtunded, that is, dulled, state or be stillborn. Now, with Pitocin, although 20 hours may not sound like a short labor, it is considerably briefer than three or four days. Babies come out healthier because they are not battering the mother's perineum for days, and the mother's perineum is not as worn and there is less likelihood of its tearing, leading to fistula formation.

All of this makes Pitocin an excellent, excellent drug, but like any other drug, it has to be used according to strict guidelines, lest it be as dangerous as giving someone too much morphine or digitalis. When Pitocin is doing too much, that is, producing too frequent or too intense contractions, it has to be cut off quickly.

LABOR

Normal labor is basically the same for everyone, although it may be experienced differently according to individual pain thresholds. In some women it begins as back pain. In others, it may be confused with indigestion. For still others, it presents itself as the worst menstrual cramps they have ever experienced; the menstrual cramp from hell surges up and the woman feels as though it is ripping out her tonsils.

After the initial stab, the pains come again every ten or fifteen or thirty minutes. That they are rhythmic and regular is what differentiates them from false labor and any other type of pain they may be mistaken for. If a contraction comes at 10:00, another at 10:20, another at 11:00, and not another until 11:40, this is not yet true labor. These wayward pains are like new recruits in the army. They do not know the cadence; they are milling around aimlessly. The muscles are saying, "We're ready. We're grown up now. We can do something," but they are not organized yet. For all the muscles and fibers to begin working together takes several hours, then suddenly the recruits fall into step and the contractions begin arriving regularly.

When the contractions are coming at the rate of one every five minutes—twelve an hour—it is time to get in touch with the physician or health care provider who is scheduled to deliver the baby. But the mother is still not in active labor, which is contractions every two to three minutes. There is no fear of the baby's arriving in the car on the way to the hospital unless the mother is one of the very, very few women who have precipitous labor. Infinitely more common is the woman who goes through contractions for many, many more hours. Prolonged labor is required because the cervix has to change in consistency from being as thick and stubby as a nose to the thinness of a sheet of paper. Imagine having a big chunk of dough and taking a rolling pin and rolling it out, then folding it and rolling it again, and again, and again, until the dough is as thin as the leaves of the most delicate French pastry. This rolling out of the cervix, called effacement, does not take place quickly; it requires many, many hours.

The thinning of the cervix is as much a measure of the progress of labor as is the dilatation of the cervix. If a mother is at six centimeters at four o'clock and the cervix is 50 percent effaced, the obstetrician may return at six o'clock to find that dilatation is still at six centimeters but now the cervix is 100 percent effaced. When that is the case, there is nothing to do but wait because these two things, dilatation and effacement, have to work together.

The contractions will just keep coming, as relentless as a blitzkrieg. The mother may plead, "Please, I need a five-minute break," but she will not be granted it. The troops—the little muscle fibers that turn the uterus into one big muscle—are on the march, and they are going to contract and contract and contract until the baby is born. The 12, 15, or 20 hours of the first stage of labor to bring the dilatation of the cervix to five centimeters is called the prodromal or latent phase. After five centimeters comes the time of maximal acceleration, the active phase of labor. The dilatation zooms up to seven, eight, nine centimeters, and the birth is well on its way. It is like watering a bamboo shoot for weeks: You keep coming back and wondering why so little is happening, then overnight it shoots up six feet. From the start of maximal acceleration (5 cm.) until the baby is born averages about six hours. This is when epidural anesthesia can be used without the risk of impeding progress, as it will do if given earlier.

Stations. The baby's head descends slowly into the mother's pelvis, coming through what are known as stations, getting closer and closer to the "exit door" and delivery. A station is the location of the bony part of the baby's head in relation to the mother's internal pelvic ischial spine; both head and spine cannot be seen by the obstetrician, only felt. The baby starts high up, at a minus three or four station. Then those Arnold Schwarzenegger muscles of the uterus start pushing the baby down, from minus three to minus two to minus one. At zero station, the baby is said to be engaged. If its head can negotiate the ischial spines at the narrowest part of the mother's pelvis and go to plus one station, it is almost certain that the baby is not too big to be delivered vaginally. After that, the stations go from plus one to plus two to plus three, and at four or five the baby is out.

When the cervix is fully dilated, the baby's head can descend into the vagina and the cervix can no longer be felt by the examiner. It behaves in the same fashion as a turtleneck sweater that first covers the head, then rolls back when the head comes through. All that the obstetrician now feels is head; the cervix is back behind the baby's head and shoulders. If the mother has been given an epidural and cannot feel the contractions, or if she is exhausted, she may not be able to push the baby out, in which case the obstetrician may use forceps or a cap with a vacuum applied to the baby's head to guide the baby out.

EPISIOTOMY

An episiotomy is a surgical incision in the vulva to allow sufficient clearance for birth. The decision to do an episiotomy cannot be made until the baby's head is really distending the vagina. Again, the clearest way to visualize it is to imagine a turtleneck sweater at the moment of greatest stretch before you yank it down and your head emerges. At this moment in the birth of a baby, whether or not to do an episiotomy is a judgment call on the part of the obstetrician. You do not want to make a cut unnecessarily, but neither do you want the baby's head suddenly to rip the tissues in a jagged, hard-to-repair fashion.

Because the baby's head is right there, the cut is made with blunt scissors rather than a scalpel. Inserting the blunt end of the scissors between the baby's head and the mother's perineum can be difficult, so you try to push the baby's head back a little, but sometimes it does not go, in which case you try to get a millimeter's leeway in the vagina. Experience helps you to judge the length of the perineum from the baby's head to the top of the anus and insert the scissors exactly far enough so that the cut is made with one quick snap of the scissors. Too long a cut and it extends into the rectum. Too short a cut and the baby's head will rip the cut through to the rectum. The average length of the cut is about an inch and a half, just enough to widen the restricting ring that is preventing the head from coming out. It is done without anesthesia because the pressure of the baby's head on the perineum has pretty well numbed it.

At this point the doctor is telling the mother, "Don't push. Don't push now. I'll let you know when," because the mother's pushing may extend the cut beyond where it should go or cause a rip in the opposite direction and suddenly there is blood gushing from the clitoris and urethra through ragged tears that are very difficult to repair. With controlled pushing, the obstetrician and the mother can work together to have her push just the right amount to get the baby out but not so much that the baby flies out like a banana from a banana peel.

The obstetrician places a towel at the mother's rectum, and in the little space for maneuvering gained by the episiotomy, gently guides the vagina over the baby's head and delivers the head. The towel is then discarded and the baby's nose and mouth suctioned before the shoulders are delivered. If the baby is being born in meconium, you do not want its initial cry, which comes when the chest is delivered, to suck that green substance into the lungs.

Often enough, you look down at the baby and see its first piece of jewelry, a necklace, which is the umbilical cord wrapped around its neck. People tend to say, "Oh, my God, the cord was wrapped around the baby's neck." If I am the one they say it to, my reply is, "So, what else is new?" because one out of every four babies has what is called a nuchal cord. The obstetrician simply pulls it over the baby's head, or if it is really snug, applies Kelly clamps in two areas, cuts the cord between the clamps, and unwraps it from the baby's neck.

THE BABY'S FIRST BREATH

The baby's nose and mouth are suctioned out with a tiny rubber "bulb" syringe as soon as the head is delivered. The shoulders and chest follow next, and since they are squeezed by the tightness of the space they are coming through, when the chest emerges from the vagina, the lungs recoil, like a fat lady getting out of a tight girdle, and that recoil pulls air into the lungs and gives the baby its first breath.

Heretofore, although the lungs have been growing and developing in utero, they have not been functioning as lungs do in air. Instead, the placenta has served as the lungs, supplying the fetus with oxygenated blood through a large vein in the umbilical cord. There are two arteries and one vein in the cord; in the reverse of the usual circulation in which arteries carry blood from the heart and veins return it to the heart, the vein in the umbilical cord carries oxygenated blood to the fetus, where it goes into the baby's belly button, through its liver, and into the right side of its heart. Two tiny arteries in the umbilical cord return the deoxygenated blood to the placenta. Thus, because the oxygen is already in the blood coming from the placenta, the baby's lungs are not needed until the moment it is born. With the baby's first breath comes the switchover from the fetal circulation to the neonatal circulation by means of physiological changes that shut down valves in the heart and open vessels to the lungs.

In a cesarean section, there is little recoil of the chest when the baby is lifted out and the residual fluid in the lungs is not squeezed out like water from a sponge, as it is when the baby travels, as nature intended, down the birth canal. Rapid, shallow breathing, known as transient tachypnea of the newborn (TTN) results. It is short-lived and the baby usually recovers without intervention.

The recoil of the chest in a vaginal birth is so automatic that the baby has to be either obtunded or severely depressed for it not to happen. The baby breathes, and when it breathes, it cries. If that first cry does not come within thirty seconds, as the obstetrician you try to be cool about it but you are waiting to hear—waiting . . . waiting. . . . You have already handed the baby off to the nurse, and now you look at her and raise your eyebrows. The nurse says, "We're having problems." You leave the mother, moving calmly so as not to alarm her or the father, and suction out the baby's nose and mouth again because the baby maybe wants to cry but there is a big blob of mucus in its nose or throat. You give it whiffs of oxygen, pat it on the back, and strike it glancingly, with a kind of slicing motion, on the soles of its feet. Hopefully, then comes "Wah!" What one used to see in the movies, the country doctor holding up the baby by the feet and smacking its bottom, is actually the worst thing you can do because spanking the baby can cause hemorrhages behind the baby's eyes.

The crying continues until the baby is soothed and comforted by being dried off and swaddled in a tight wrap; it has spent its life so far in a small space and being confined reassures it. The crying has let you know the lungs are functioning, and a pink face and chest verify that the tissues are being perfused with oxygen. Blue fingertips and toenails are not alarming, but if the baby is blue all over, that indicates trouble. The color is not a cerulean or cobalt blue but a dusky shade, only visible in bright light. You say to yourself, "This kid is not pinking up," and you quickly undertake resuscitative procedures.

THE BABY'S ARRIVAL

People sometimes comment, "Dr. Thornton, you have a strong handshake," and I tell them I ought to, I've been pulling out babies for 25 years. The baby comes out and you have to quickly get a grip on it between the neck and the shoulders, not a viselike grip but firm enough, like a running back holding a football, so there is no chance of it slipping through your fingers. With the baby lying on your arm, you turn your forearm toward your body so you can suction the baby's nose and mouth again. You really need a good degree of manual dexterity because the baby is slippery and crying, and you are holding it on one arm while you get ready to cut the cord with the other hand. You allow some of the blood in the cord to go into the baby because it is good oxygen, and you wait for the pulsations to stop, then you clamp the cord and cut it.

The mother may be saying, "I want the baby on my chest. I want the bonding to start now," but the baby needs to go over to the warmer, which has radiant heat coming from overhead. It has just come from a mother whose internal temperature is 99.7 degrees into a room that is 75 degrees, and that is a shock to it. The nurse puts the baby's head down so all the fluid drains and the last of it can be sucked out, enabling the lungs to handle the blood that is now being pumped to them. When the baby is breathing well on its own, the nurse wraps it up and puts a little cap on its head because, like adults, it loses body warmth mostly through its head. After all this is done is time enough to be concerned about bonding.

When I first heard about the Leboyer method of dim lights and music and warm water to put the baby in, I thought it sounded great—until it became clear that babies did not do as well because we could not see whether the blood was perfusing their little extremities. A baby's hands and feet need to be pink, but if they were blue and it was not noticed for 15 minutes in the dim light, they were not intubated and given oxygen as promptly as they should have been.

Bonding. Granted that there is such an entity as bonding, I really do not believe it must occur in the first minutes of life. In the 1970s the dictum was put forward that "you need to bond in the first five minutes, you need to have eye contact, or else you are going to be a bad parent." Nonsense. Think of the mothers who adopt children. Think of the mothers who have cesarean sections and are under anesthesia for the first five minutes. They certainly bond with their children just as firmly, just as unbreakably, as the mother who has the baby on her breast immediately after birth. The first imperative is to make sure the baby is healthy enough to bond.

The mother as well as the baby may be cold, shivering with what are called the postpartum shakes. It can be quite frightening, leading the mother to believe that she is going into an epileptic seizure, but it is a natural reaction. The placenta is a heat-retaining organ; after it is delivered, that source of heat is gone and the mother's thermostat is trying to readjust. Until it does, she shivers, which is why there are warm blankets in the delivery room.

APGAR SCORES

Dr. Virginia Apgar was an anesthesiologist at Columbia Presbyterian Medical Center where I trained. I never met her, but I knew her through my mentor, the late Dr. L. Stanley James, who had worked with her. As an anesthesiologist called on to intubate newborns who were in trouble, it occurred to Dr. Apgar that it would be useful to establish objective standards for when resuscitative measures were indicated and when they were not needed. Accordingly, she developed what came to be known as the Apgar score. It is not meant to be a measure of whether the child will grow up to go to Harvard or, contrariwise, whether he or she will have a learning disability. All it tells is whether or not the baby requires resuscitative measures within the first five minutes after it is born.

There are five parameters to the Apgar score: heart rate, respirations, muscle tone, skin color, and the grimace. Each is scored zero, one, or two, and the scoring is done at one minute and five minutes, sometimes at ten minutes, after the baby is born, usually by the circulating nurse—never by the obstetrician because the observer needs to be objective. Heart rate is the first category. If there is no heartbeat, the score is zero. Below 100 beats per minute, the score is one; over 100 beats, two. Concerning respiration, if the baby is not breathing, the score is zero; if its breathing is irregular and slow, one; if it is crying lustily, two. The next category is muscle tone. If the baby is flaccid, if it lies there like a wet noodle, the Apgar score, as you can imagine, is zero. With some flexion of the extremities, some faint movement, the score goes to one. With active motion, it becomes a two. The fourth category is skin color. Blue is scored zero. If the baby's body is pink but the fingers and toes are still kind of blue and pale, that rates a one; if everything is pink, that is a two. The fifth category deals with reflex irritability. No response to the catheter when it is placed in the baby's nose is zero, a slight response is one, a grimace is two.

The numbers are added together, with ten being a perfect score. Few babies are a ten at one minute because a baby has been in utero with the placenta acting as its lungs and now it has to shift over to its own lungs to supply oxygen to the extremities. In one minute the blood may get to everything except the hands and feet, which are farthest from the heart and which tend to be blue with what is called acrocyanosis. In five minutes the extremities have pinkened, and the five-minute Apgar score goes up to ten. Or it may be nine or eight, and that is still fine.

A one-minute Apgar score of zero to three indicates a severely depressed baby who needs to be intubated to get oxygen into its lungs and given epinephrine to stimulate its heart; this is a CPR emergency. With an Apgar score of three to seven, a baby is moderately depressed and needs to have a little bit of oxygen and some stimulation, like the rubbing of its back. Any score above seven means the baby is okay. At five minutes, if the Apgar score is still below seven, a neonatalogist—a highly trained specialist in the care of newborns—is summoned, and an umbilical artery catheter is readied for the infusion of medication.

Actually, the neonatologist on duty is called in before the baby is born if the obstetrician spots any indication that the baby is going to be in trouble. The monitor may indicate that the baby's heart rate is crashing, and/or when the membranes were ruptured, meconium as thick and green as pea soup came out. When there are such indications, as soon as the baby is out, boom! five people are on top of the kid, working on it. That is why we have good babies. In the old days general practitioners delivered the babies and they were not aggressive. They did not measure the blood gases. Kids today are smarter than when I was a baby because we make sure there is oxygen going to the brain.

If the hospital does not have an in-house neonatalogist on call, the newborn in trouble has to be transported to a facility with a neonatal intensive care unit, and time is the enemy, always the enemy, in obstetrics and neonatalogy. I have no wish to denigrate community hospitals or midwives, but if a woman really values the whole experience, from conception until she takes the baby home, and she does not want to take any chances, she will seek care with specialists and in facilities that are prepared to deal immediately with the unpredictable. (See chapter 14.)

THE OBSTETRICIAN AND THE NEONATOLOGIST

The obstetrician suctions the baby's nose and mouth as soon as the head is delivered, but after the baby is born and the cord is cut, the baby is handed off to the nurse or pediatrician or, if there has been reason to have one standing by, the neonatologist. The nurse is trained in estimating Apgar scores, and if at one minute, the score is low, she hits a light signal and the neonatologist is there before the next four minutes go by.

While the neonatologist is resuscitating the baby, the obstetrician stays with the mother. The placenta has yet to come out; there may be bleeding, and she must be watched for signs of hemorrhage or difficulty in breathing. But if there is no help at hand and the baby is in trouble, the obstetrician tries quickly to stabilize the mother, clamp the placenta off and leave it in, and then go to the baby, on the way grabbing up a kit containing endotracheal tubes, nasotracheal tubes, catheters, epinephrine, sodium bicarbonate, and AMBU-bags (AMBU stands for "assisted manual breathing unit").

If the baby is grunting and you see retractions in its chest, its lungs are not functioning as they should. You have to get the airway open, and you have to maintain the baby's circulation. With a laryngoscope in the baby's mouth, you visualize the baby's vocal cords and thread a catheter through the baby's windpipe, either to suction out mucus or meconium or to administer oxygen to the lungs. It takes a great deal of experience to know how much oxygen to administer, and even in the best of hands, resuscitative efforts can force too much oxygen into the lungs, causing them to collapse. If the oxygen does not revive the baby, time is of the essence and the baby is given a little shot of epinephrine in the heart. Next comes the threading of a catheter into the umbilical artery. The artery is about the size of number 9 spaghetti, and to get a catheter into that takes skill. What goes through the catheter is sodium bicarbonate.

If you are a runner, you are aware that when there is not much oxygen left in your muscles, you go to anaerobic circulation and get cramps because of the lactic acid buildup in the muscles. The same thing happens in the newborn: If not enough oxygen is getting to the muscles, the baby's body is trying to get energy without oxygen and that leads to an increase in lactic acid. Because a high level of lactic acid is not good for the heart muscle, which can go into cardiac arrest, the acid needs to be neutralized with sodium bicarbonate. The neonatalogist or obstetrician works back and forth, giving whiffs of oxygen and administering small increments of sodium bicarbonate and other medications until the baby is stabilized.

Sometimes a father in the labor room says, "I didn't see you pick up the baby and smack it on the back. If you did that, it would probably be breathing now." Five or ten minutes then go into educating the father to persuade him that you really have not failed to do the best possible thing for his baby.

It also happens that people, especially attorneys, use the Apgar score in ways that were not intended. For instance, the baby may later be found to have some neurological deficit, and the attorney says, "The Apgar scores were one and five, so the cerebral palsy was caused by birth trauma." That conclusion cannot be justified on the basis of the Apgar scores alone. The same is true for the use of Apgar scores for nursery school admission. It is like saying the child had a D in third grade so he or she can never go to college. The Apgar score applies only to the first five minutes of life and is intended only to define the status of the baby for the obstetrician, nurses, and pediatrician so that they know what, if anything, needs to be done to ensure the survival and health of the baby.

In addition to calling out the Apgar scores at one and five minutes, the circulating nurse is responsible for immediately taking the baby's footprints and putting tags on all its extremities to identify it as this mother's baby. If either the mother or the baby has a problem, the nurse hits a button, a light goes on in the nurses' station, and people come. Or the obstetrician simply summons help. There is a lot of traffic in and around delivery rooms. I have never called for assistance and not had help arrive.

THE THIRD STAGE OF LABOR

There are three stages of labor, the first being from the start of contractions until the cervix is fully dilated and the second from then until the time of delivery. The third stage of labor is from the time the baby is delivered until delivery of the placenta, no more than 30 minutes. While waiting for delivery of the placenta, the obstetrician collects a sample of blood from the umbilical cord, now separated from the baby, so that it can be checked to determine the blood type and Rh status of the baby. The vessels of the umbilical cord are also examined to make sure that there is one vein and two arteries. If there is just one artery, the absence is important because it can be associated with bladder and kidney problems in the baby. The pediatrician or the nursery must be told about this finding so that a close watch can be kept on the baby. As for the excess cord on the baby, the nurse cuts it and places a plastic clamp on it close to the point where it is attached to the baby's abdomen. The clamp can be removed in two or three days or allowed to fall off with the cord.

Then the obstetrician waits for the placenta to come out. There is no question of tugging on it because that can turn the uterus inside out and send the mother into shock. The uterus must be left alone to do what it is supposed to do, which is to shut down the blood supply to the placenta and expel it. The mother is surprised that she is still having contractions, but it is the contractions that accomplish what remains to be done.

After the placenta is delivered, Pitocin is started in tiny amounts to prompt the uterus to continue its contractions. The uterus needs to clamp down like a balled fist because it is this clamping that controls bleeding from the raw edges of the uterus where the placenta was attached. Interestingly, women with blood dyscrasias or clotting platelet abnormalities do not have any particular problem with bleeding after childbirth because it is not the clotting factors in the blood that stop the bleeding in this circumstance but the tourniquet action of the contracted uterus on the blood vessels.

What is called a boggy uterus, or uterine atony, is the failure of the uterus to clamp down. The blood just keeps coming and coming. The blood vessels course through the muscles, the myofibrils, in the uterus, and unless the muscles clamp down the blood is going to keep flowing. A nurse is often recruited to massage the mother's abdomen to persuade the uterine muscles to clamp down. If ordinary massage does not work, the cry goes out: "Get the biggest nurse around! Send Brunhilda in here to do the massaging!" Hopefully, with vigorous massage the uterus becomes like a hard rubber ball and the bleeding stops.

If it does not, more Pitocin is given, along with methergine, a medication administered intravenously that causes blood vessel constriction. If the bleeding still continues, F2 alpha, prostaglandin type, is injected directly into the uterus. Some practitioners believe in packing the uterus through the vagina and cervix—as though they were stuffing a turkey—with about 50 yards of sterile gauze in an attempt to stop the bleeding. But packing distends the uterus and may hide the fact that the bleeding is still going on. By the time all the packing has been soaked through and it becomes obvious the bleeding has not stopped, the patient has lost unaffordable amounts of blood.

If all measures fail and the uterus is still like a floppy bag and the blood is still flowing, the only thing to be done is to whisk the patient to the operating room for a life-saving hysterectomy. Every minute 500 cc. of blood course through the uterus. That is a pint of blood, and with only 12 pints of blood in the entire body, there is not much leeway as far as time is concerned. You tell the parents this and ask them to sign a consent form.

The parents are shocked. Their reaction is: "It can't be. We just had a little baby. Everything's over. The baby's fine." The usual books have not told them about this eventuality. You warn them there cannot be any delay, but suddenly one of the parents is saying, "No, I don't want to sign." You think "Oh, geez," and you go through the whole explanation again. They have to sign, the hysterectomy has to be done or else the mother will bleed to death, but it takes the parents awhile to snap out of their denial and register the seriousness of the situation.

Hemorrhage that cannot be stopped is one of the problematic aspects of a home delivery. The mother delivers and everyone is hanging over the baby but then the attendant comes back and the bed is soaked with blood, she massages the uterus like mad, and a few minutes later she calls 911, but by then it is too late.

EPISIOTOMY REPAIR

After the placenta has been delivered and the uterus has clamped down, the obstetrician examines the cervix and the side walls of the vagina to check for lacerations. This is an instance in which strong lighting is needed because it is like peering into a Campbell's tomato soup can. Right after delivery the cervix looks like a thinned out piece of liver. It is a floppy thing but already beginning to firm up, and in four weeks, at the postpartum checkup, it will have returned to normal.

After checking thoroughly for lacerations, if there has been an episiotomy, it is repaired. Some doctors do the repair while waiting for the placenta to come out, but this is not good practice because the vagina, after it has been repaired, is once again a small orifice, and the placenta, which is about the size of a large grapefruit, can disrupt the stitches. It is essential that the episiotomy be sewn up very carefully because the tunnel of the vagina and down by the rectum has been cut to spread the tissues open for the passage of the baby, and the area must be put back together again. If the cut has gone into the rectum and it is not repaired properly, fecal incontinence may result.

Surgical training is needed to accomplish the repair skillfully enough so that the patient is not left with residual problems. Knowing this, some midwives, although they can do episiotomies, would prefer not to and go to some lengths to avoid them. They say, "We'll just iron out the perineum, iron it out with lavender oil." But the perineum can be ironed out just so much before it hits the breaking point and rips.

One night I was called in for a patient of a type I have come to recognize, the sort of woman who is wearing a mask over her eyes and saying, "I don't want an episiotomy. Don't cut me." Since I did not want to come on like an overbearing obstetrician, against my better judgment I just kept ironing and ironing the perineum, and . . . pop! The baby's head came out and ripped up everything. It was exactly what I tell my medical students must never be allowed to happen. It looked like a grenade had gone off in this lady's perineum. There were lacerations all the way up the vagina to the cervix, in the front to the clitoris, in the back to and through the rectum. The doula, the person in midwifery who accompanies the laboring patient, was cooing over the baby with the parents, taking no notice of this battlefield that had to be repaired. Again and again I had to ask for more suture material, and while I stitched, I kicked myself because this should not have happened. One of my professors used to say, "Never give the patient an even break because you'll be taking counsel from an incompetent person," and he was right. The patient was not trained to deliver babies; I was; and I should not have let her have her way. But I did, and no good deed goes unpunished; it took me an hour and a half to repair the damage.

Even under the best of circumstances, an episiotomy repair is a tricky business because the tissues are torn and ripped and swollen and filled with blood; they have been traumatized for hours, and it is like putting a needle into butter because they are so fragile and friable. If the patient has had epidural anesthesia and it is still functioning, the amount of anesthetic is increased so that she does not feel the suturing; otherwise, a local anesthetic is used. This procedure is also tricky. You need to know exactly how much of the anesthetic to use and where to put it because lidocaine toxicity is a possibility. If the mother starts talking and rapidly becomes garrulous, you know she is having a reaction to the anesthetic.

THE FATHER IN THE DELIVERY ROOM

It used to be that nobody was in the delivery room but the mother, the doctor, and the trained nurse. But now the father is there too. In the way. Asking questions. You try to be understanding because you know he wants to be part of his child's arrival in the world, but sometimes you have to say, "I understand where you are coming from, but right now, it would really help if you would sit down and shut up." Perhaps it is nervousness but some men talk and talk, asking, "Doctor, what's this? What's that?" They do not realize that you are trying to listen to parameters that may be very subtle, that all your concentration is on returning a live wife and healthy baby to him.

Not surprisingly, some men faint in the delivery room, in which case the nurse has to abandon whatever she is doing to give the father spirits of ammonia and check to see whether he has cut himself or banged his head when he fell. People tend to have a fairy-tale view of the birth of a baby, perhaps garnered from the movies, and men look forward to witnessing the mystery of birth, only to discover that it is not what they thought it was going to be. The wife the man knows so well is not the same person; she is in pain and screaming and yelling. She may be defecating or urinating on herself; there is blood; she has monitors hanging out of her vagina. It is not a pretty sight. Very soon the husband may be saying, "Can't you do a cesarean right now?" because he wants to get the ordeal over with. And, indeed, three hours later we may have to do a cesarean, but that comes only after we have exhausted all the avenues of a natural birth. The husband, not understanding that, yells, "I told you three hours ago to do a cesarean!" and perhaps forevermore believes the obstetrician is a sadist who enjoys making women suffer.

Somehow—I am not sure how—obstetrics has come to be considered a family affair. Of all the medical and surgical procedures, only obstetrics is asked to go against the tenets and principles of asepsis. People would not expect to be present in the operating room if a woman was having her gallbladder out, but in some birthing centers, even the children in the family are allowed to be present to touch the baby's head as it is coming out. The more people in the room, the greater the danger of infection, particularly if an episiotomy must be done. This is a surgical procedure, and the atmosphere should be as free as possible of the bacteria in people's noses and mouths and on their hands. In short, I believe we have become all too chummy about the birthing process and that a return to a more rigorous atmosphere is in order.

LDRP ROOMS

The latest thing in hospitals is LDRP rooms in which Labor, Delivery, Recovery, and the Postpartum stay all take place in one room. The room tends to be handsomely decorated in order to persuade women that they are getting a good deal, but the real reason for LDRP rooms is that it is more cost-effective to have one room for one patient versus a labor suite, delivery room, recovery room, and postpartum floor. Even though in the LDRP the mahogany armoire concealing the medical equipment is beautiful, I would rather the emphasis was on functionality. Ask where the cesarean section room is and you are likely to be told, "Go down the hall to the second intersection, hang a left, and it is at the end of the next corridor one flight down," when really it should be right next to the LDRP rooms where you can get to it in a really big hurry when you need to.

Another concern I have is whether the room is cleaned as

thoroughly as a delivery room is, whether we are any longer observing the strict asepsis that used to be the rule. We have become so cavalier about the use of antibiotics that we have forgotten that maternal infection can be a very real problem. I would venture to predict that if we continue to disregard the possibility, we will see it return as tuberculosis has. Delivery is a messy business, what with the blood and the placenta; it is really a semisurgical procedure that ought to take place in a sterile environment that is thoroughly disinfected after the patient has been moved to another area.

When LDRP rooms first came in, I soured on them because the lighting was such that the obstetrician could not see the vagina and lacerations went unnoticed until the patient perhaps returned to the hospital with hematomas and such. Although the lighting has been improved, I still believe it is preferable for labor to take place in one room, delivery in another, and after that for the patient to be moved to a pleasant postpartum area. But we are at the mercy of space-allotment committees, architects, and engineers who talk about promoting bonding and love but are really into cost-cutting and efficiency.

Hospitals bank on the fact that for the majority of deliveries special equipment will not be needed, but I like to proceed on a worst-case scenario. I want to be able to put out my hand and instantly pick up the right instrument. I want to be able to say, "Drop the table. Let's get the baby out now!" I do not want to have to wait until the bed is maneuvered out the door, down the hall, down another corridor, into an elevator, and into the cesarean section room. Pregnant patients checking out a hospital will be shown the rocking chair and the colorful curtains, but what they really should be asking is: Will the bed fit through the door, and how far away is the cesarean section room?

THE FOURTH STAGE

The fourth stage of delivery is from the time of the delivery of the placenta until one hour later. After 20 or so hours of labor, after further contractions to expel the placenta and have the uterus tighten, after the surgical repair, the mother is exhausted, which is why I take issue with the childbirth-preparation classes that make the mother believe: "I want the baby on my breast. I want it to breast-feed. I want the bonding to begin immediately." That mother has been through labor as hard as 20 hours of cracking rocks at Leavenworth, with no time off, no lunch breaks, with every two or three minutes feeling as though she has been prodded by a stun gun. Having the baby on her abdomen may be the last thing she wants, but she feels guilty because she has been told what she is supposed to feel. Although a few rare mothers will say they want to breast-feed, they are women having a second or third child. The first-time mother usually whispers, "Is it all right if the nurse takes the baby, Dr. Thornton? I'm done in." I say, "Sure, sure, it's the sensible thing to do."

And it is. The mother needs a rest. The baby needs a rest. I need a rest. We have been through a lot together.

POSTPARTUM CHECKUP

After childbirth the mother's body goes through some major reparative changes. The uterus is returning to its nonpregnant size by contracting down (involuting), causing a bloody discharge called lochia, which is normal. Initially, lochia is bright red, like a period, but over several weeks the color gets lighter, and at four to six weeks postpartum it ends altogether. Uterine cramping may be present during this involution process.

Another very common but little known change that occurs right after delivery is dramatic swelling of the feet and lower extremities. This is due to the natural fluid shifts occurring in the body after delivery. Since the feet and ankles are the lowest parts of the body, fluid tends to accumulate in them, but with continued urination the swelling disappears and the new mother can once again fit into her slippers.

A postpartum checkup by the obstetrician is scheduled four to six weeks after delivery. The patient is examined for any infection, and if an episiotomy was performed, to make certain that it is healing properly. A blood sample is drawn to check for anemia. A thyroid function test, although not routine, is desirable because the pregnancy may have triggered the gland to become hyperactive. Contraceptive methods are discussed, and if the patient decides to go on the Pill, cholesterol levels and a liver function test are ordered as baseline studies. Patients are often asked not to engage in sexual intercourse prior to the postpartum visit because their contraceptive methods may not be effective and they can become pregnant again.

POINTS TO REMEMBER

- The average female pelvis is gynecoid in shape, just right for a baby to scoot through.
- A cephalopelvic disproportion between the fetal head and the maternal pelvis may necessitate a cesarean section.
- The amniotic sac, or "bag of waters," is a thin membrane inside the uterus filled with the amniotic fluid in which the fetus lives.
- If the amniotic membrane ruptures prematurely, 80 percent of mothers deliver within seven days.
- During labor, external and internal monitors allow a careful and continuing check on the status of both mother and child.
- Pitocin, a synthetic version of the hormone that prompts uterine contractions, speeds up labor.
- Rhythmic and regular contractions are the hallmark of labor.
- Active labor is contractions every two or three minutes.
- In labor the cervix has to change from being thick and stubby to the thinness of a sheet of paper in a process called effacement.
- An episiotomy is a surgical incision in the vulva to allow sufficient room for the baby's head to come through.
- The baby's Apgar scores are used to indicate whether there is a need to resuscitate the newborn. They are not a measure to predict future intelligence.
- Delivery of the placenta usually takes place within 30 minutes after the birth of the baby.
- Failure of the uterus to contract and shut off excessive postpartum bleeding rapidly becomes an emergency situation.
- Painstaking repair of an episiotomy obviates future health problems for the mother.

12

CESAREAN SECTION

∽

FETAL MONITORING • STAT SECTION • FETAL DISTRESS • ATTEMPT AT VAGINAL DELIVERY FOLLOWED BY A CESAREAN • VAGINAL BIRTH AFTER CESAREAN (VBAC) • DELIVERY OF PREMATURE BABIES • AGE OF THE FETUS •

One of the hallowed bits of knowledge everyone possesses, but which happens not to be true, is that a cesarean section is so called because Julius Caesar entered the world by this means. In Roman times, however, a mother's body was cut open to deliver the baby only if the mother was already dead—it was a postmortem procedure to save the baby—and Caesar's mother happened, as we know, to have outlived her son by many years. Thus, Caesar's birth must have taken place by the customary route, and the more likely derivation of cesarean is that it comes from the Latin *caedere*, "to cut."

FETAL MONITORING

In a cesarean section, an incision is made through the abdominal and uterine walls to deliver the baby. Until recently, the reason for performing a cesarean was because the baby was too big to be delivered vaginally. The mother would labor for hours and hours and hours, to the point of total exhaustion, until it became obvious that her bony pelvis was not going to accommodate a baby of the size waiting to be born. This is still a prime reason for doing a section—difficult and prolonged labor accounts for 30 percent of all cesareans—but now it is far from the only reason. Breech presentation is the reason in 12 percent of cases and fetal distress in 9 percent; other reasons include twins and mothers with toxemia, diabetes, or ruptured membranes.

During labor, the strength of the mother's contractions and the condition of the baby are tracked by internal and external monitors. The external monitors include a Doppler, to register the fetal heart rate, and a tokodynamometer, which is a strap placed on the mother's abdomen; each contraction registers on the strap, indicating the event but not its degree of intensity. These external monitors are useful but not nearly as informative as the internal monitors: an electrode placed on the baby's scalp to register the fetal heart rate and a catheter threaded into the uterus to measure the intensity of the contractions.

There is some controversy over whether every woman in labor needs the electronic monitors, a main argument being why cannot a nurse just listen to the fetal heart every ten minutes with a stethoscope? He or she can, but the nurse may also be taking care of two or three patients, may need to go on a break, or may go off duty with a change of shifts, and the necessary check every ten minutes does not get done. The beauty of electronic monitoring is that all it does is count. It does not go to the bathroom, it does not get called away, and it does not have to make decisions. Electronic monitors are a boon and have saved many lives.

Unfortunately, they have not significantly reduced the incidence of cerebral palsy, which is what prompted their initial introduction. Although it is not known what causes cerebral palsy, it appears now that it is less frequently caused by birth trauma than by some neurological derangement in the development of the brain during pregnancy. On the positive side, thanks to electronic monitoring, we do not see intrapartum deaths anymore, something I witnessed a lot when I was in training. A patient checked into the hospital, was examined, and it was verified that she was in labor; the doctor would go off and return an hour later to find there was no fetal heartbeat. The baby had died because, without monitoring, the subtle signs that it was in trouble were missed. A baby has no way of communicating with the outside world: It cannot call out, "My heart rate is fine. Everything's cool. Leave me alone," or "Get me out of here. I can't breathe. There's no oxygen in here." But now we have the monitor on the baby's scalp to tell us there are late decelerations in the heart rate or no variability, signs that the baby is in distress and needs to be rescued.

I have practiced in two worlds, the time before electronic monitoring and the time after, and I can say without a shadow of a doubt that babies are stronger and better now, healthier, brighter, and more intelligent because at the first sign they are in trouble, we go in and deliver them, either by forceps or cesarean section. Some people object to electronic monitoring on the basis that it is invasive, but I think it is absolutely indispensable and, as far as I am aware, without a downside. Perhaps if the mother has herpes or a lesion of some sort, there may be some possibility of transmitting an infection to the baby's head, but that must be very, very rare. Every year four million babies are born in this country and monitoring has been going on for thirty years; if it was in any way deleterious, the drawbacks would have declared themselves by now.

STAT SECTION

An elective cesarean section is one that has been scheduled in advance because the baby is breech or the mother has diabetes or high blood pressure. A stat section, in contrast, is an emergency procedure done because the baby is showing signs of fetal distress. Stat is from the Latin *statim*, "immediately." Recently a husband said to me, "Okay, get this over with stat," and when I asked where he had learned that, he answered, "The television show *ER*. I knew it meant in a hurry because as soon as they said that everybody started running in and doing something."

It is perfectly true that when a stat section is called for, you do not fool around; you move fast. According to the American College of Obstetricians and Gynecologists, a woman in labor should be in a setting where the lapsed time from decision to incision is no more than 30 minutes. Usually the holdup is anesthesia, not the incision. In smaller hospitals there may not be an obstetrical anesthesiologist on duty 24 hours a day; if only one anesthesiologist is covering the operating room, he or she may be in the midst of an emergency elsewhere when needed in the delivery room.

If an epidural is running, we give the patient a bolus—a large shot—of the anesthetic, wait until she cannot feel, and then go in. But often we cannot wait for that big shot of anesthetic to take effect sufficiently for major surgery to be carried out, so we say to the anesthetist, "Put her out. I've got to get in here!" That means an inhalant anesthetic and intubation with an endotracheal tube to the lungs. If the woman were not pregnant, the anesthesiologist would have the option not to intubate, but because of changes in the gastric emptying time of the stomach, a pregnant woman is always considered to have a full stomach even though she has not eaten in a day. With a full stomach, she may vomit and have the stomach contents get into her lungs.

From the time the woman is unconscious and I can start operating until I get the baby out is one minute. Literally one minute, unless I encounter adhesions or blood vessels in places they have no business being or the woman is very heavy and there are many layers to go through. I remember an occasion where the baby's heart rate was flat, an agonal tracing—agonal meaning the moment before death—and the instant the anesthesiologist said "Yes!" I cut through all the layers with one sweep of the knife and had the baby out of there. Had that sweep been in the wrong place, I would have gotten the baby out but the mother would have been bleeding to death from lacerated uterine arteries. Not to get it in the wrong place is the reason for four years of obstetrical training.

The baby lived. And that is almost always the way it turns out because, as a perinatalogist, I am watching for signs so subtle that other people may miss them. The nurse may say, "Why did you do a stat section? The baby came out okay." But that is just the point—to have the baby come out okay. You do not want babies that are not breathing or have no heart rate. The trick is to go in immediately when you see a change, to get in and get the baby out quickly so that it can have ventilatory assistance and be resuscitated.

Every cesarean that is not elective is not necessarily a stat section. For instance, if a woman is stuck at six centimeters, we will decide to do a cesarean, but there is no tearing hurry. We only do stat sections if the fetal heart rate is problematic. Almost never is it for the mother; basically, it is for fetal distress.

FETAL DISTRESS

Fetal distress can take many forms, but essentially what we are talking about is the heart rate of the fetus, which is the only parameter we are really looking at in labor. The obstetrician reads the strip from the fetal monitor, which is like looking at an EKG or an EEG, and learns from it not just the heart rate but the configuration of the heart rate. The heart rate may be within the normal range of 120 to 160, but if the line is flat enough to write your name on, you immediately ask why there is no variability, no little spikes. Perhaps the mother has been given Demerol for the pain of the contractions; she may be having epidural anesthesia; or the baby may be in a sleep cycle of 20 to 40 minutes during which there is decreased variability. Or—and this is the main concern—the baby may not be getting enough oxygen. Lack of oxygen affects the heart muscle of the baby and flattens out the variability on the strip.

If the mother was not given Demerol and she is not receiving epidural anesthesia, and if 40 minutes have gone by and the baby should be out of a sleep cycle but the tracing is still flat and the mother is only at four centimeters, what do you do? Time was, you would assume fetal distress and go to a cesarean, but now what we do is take a drop of blood from the baby's head and analyze it to determine the pH. In a fetus the pH should be between 7.25 and 7.35, starting out at the beginning of labor at the high of 7.35, then going down because of the stress of labor (long labors hurt babies too). If the pH drops into a more and more acidotic range, this means the oxygen reserve is being depleted. As discussed earlier in this chapter, just as runners who have used up their oxygen reserves go into anaerobic metabolism and lactic acid builds up in their muscles, so does lactic acid build up in the fetus. The lactic acid affects the blood gases and sends the pH reading down toward the acid range. If the drop of blood taken from the baby gives a reading of 7.27, okay, fine, it is in the normal range; the baby has enough oxygen. But if the pH is 7.22, I begin to get nervous. Below 7.20, I go for a stat section. The baby has to be delivered really quickly because its oxygen supply is too low.

If labor has not progressed very far, the cervix is still closed, and you cannot get to the baby to take a droplet of blood, it is a judgment call whether or not to do a cesarean when the heart rate is normal but the pattern is abnormal. You wait an hour, but then you say, "We can't take a chance. We have to do a section."

The ability to recognize and electronically monitor fetal distress is the reason we no longer have babies dying during labor.

ATTEMPT AT VAGINAL DELIVERY FOLLOWED BY A CESAREAN

The normal course of labor and delivery does not follow a script for an *I Love Lucy* show in which Lucy suddenly blurts, "Oh, I'm having contractions!" and after the commercial, she is in the delivery room and has the baby. The average time for the first half of labor from the start of contractions until the active phase when the cervix is dilated four or five centimeters is 20 hours. After that, the cervix should dilate approximately 1.2 centimeters an hour in a woman who is having her first child, 1.5 centimeters an hour in a woman who has had a child or children previously. This means that if the patient is at 5 centimeters at four o'clock in the afternoon, at six o'clock the cervix should be at 7 centimeters, by 8 o'clock at 9 centimeters, and by 10 o'clock she should be fully dilated and ready to deliver. This progression is called the Friedman curve; if the patient deviates from it, the obstetrician must decide whether to do a cesarean section.

Say the patient is at 6 centimeters at four o'clock in the afternoon. The obstetrician figures, "Okay, I'm going to be out of here by midnight." But when he or she returns at six o'clock, the patient, instead of being at 8 centimeters, is still at 6 centimeters. It has to be for one of two reasons: Either her contractions are not strong enough or the baby is too big for the size of her pelvis. The first thing the obstetrician does is ascertain whether the patient is having effective contractions by checking the tracing on the uterine monitor. If the monitor indicates strong contractions every two or three minutes for the previous two hours but the patient is still at 6 centimeters, her body is saying it is not going to be able to deliver this baby.

Birth is made possible by the mother and baby working together—the maternal-fetal unit of her bony pelvis and the baby's head negotiating through it. The baby's skull bones are not fixed and fused like an adult's; they slide like overlapping plates as the baby's head leads the way through the maternal pelvis. Sometimes the plates slide and slide and the head gets to the smallest possible diameter and it still will not fit through the pelvis. The baby's head becomes swollen because the mother is pushing and pushing and pushing and the soft tissue of the baby's head is taking a beating. The baby, if it comes out then, is a little swollen-headed, conehead kid. If it does not come out,

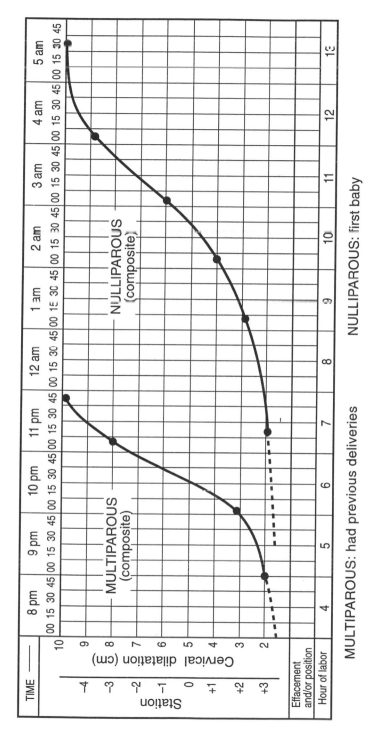

MULTIPAROUS: had previous deliveries   NULLIPAROUS: first baby

The Friedman (Labor) Curve

either the mother or the baby or both are at risk of serious complications unless something is done.

In an industrialized country like the United States, a cesarean section at this point is routine, but in underdeveloped countries where women deliver far from a hospital, mother and child fairly often lose their lives. The mother tries, the baby tries, but they cannot manage together to get the baby into the world. The baby's head looks like a banana when the dead fetus is taken out of the mother, and she has died because, with hour after hour after hour of contractions ramming the baby's head against the soft tissue of her bladder and rectum, the tissue becomes thin and separates and she bleeds to death. In this country the national mortality rate is 7 or 8 per 100,000 births, but in other parts of the world it is as high as 200 or 300, even 400, per 100,000 births.

We obstetricians think the mortality rate in childbirth is still too high in this country. We do not want to lose a single baby or mother, which is why we do not hesitate to do a cesarean section if labor threatens to go on too long. The pounding on the mother's soft tissues can be so remorseless that it results in fistula formation—an opening between the vagina and the rectum or bladder. This compromises her quality of life and future ability to have children, and the baby is also endangered because with each contraction there is a decrease in the amount of oxygen reaching it.

However, a cesarean section is not always the answer. To return to the example of the patient who is at 6 centimeters at four o'clock and still at 6 centimeters at six o'clock, the obstetrician may look at the monitors and discover that the contractions are piddling ones, strong enough to carry labor this far but not strong enough to go the rest of the way. The mother says, "I'm trying, I'm trying," but obviously something more is needed. This is when the obstetrician calls for Pitocin. Pitocin is administered in tiny doses, milliunit by milliunit, by an electronic machine that drips it into a vein very, very slowly. The reason for the slowness is that large doses of Pitocin may not only cause the uterus to contract too much but also cause fluid retention, resulting in water overload in the mother.

The obstetrician watches to see the effect of the Pitocin, whether the intensity of the contractions increases to at least 50 millimeters of mercury on the internal monitor. The external monitor that the mother has on her abdomen only indicates when a contraction occurs, not its intensity. The residents that I train often try to duck out of placing an internal fetal monitor because it is a somewhat involved procedure. However, if you have been relying only on the external monitor and the patient stays at six centimeters, you have no idea of the actual intensity of the contractions and will need to insert an internal monitor and wait for two more hours to find out what is happening; whereas if the monitor has been in place all along, you can review the strip and immediately see the strength of the contractions during the previous two hours. If the strip shows solid contractions, the patient needs a cesarean section without delay, but if the tracing is like little anthills rather than camel humps, Pitocin is needed. After the Pitocin is started and the tracing shows strong contractions but the cervix remains at 6 centimeters, a cesarean section is needed. On the other hand, if the cervix goes to 8 centimeters, or, indeed, shows any degree of change, we ride with it; we keep going until we know for certain that there is no chance for a natural birth.

Meanwhile, the husband may be beating the obstetrician over the head, yelling, "My wife's in pain! Cut her! I've never seen her like this! You'd better cut her!"

When I am the one being beaten, I can only explain that all possibility of a natural delivery has to be exhausted before surgery is undertaken because the risk of such complications as infection and bleeding is eight to ten times greater with a cesarean than with a vaginal delivery. As I noted earlier, the word obstetrics is derived from a Greek word meaning "to stand by." If the monitor tells us the baby is too big, we know we are justified in going in. Or if the monitor shows that the baby's heartbeat, which is normally between 120 and 160, stays below 100 or goes much over 160, then we know the child has fetal distress and has to be gotten out of there. But otherwise we wait.

Not every obstetrician is content to wait. A woman entering the hospital at one or two centimeters still has a long way to go, but the occasional doctor will say after three hours, "She's had her trial of labor. Let's do a c-section." But three hours is not a long enough trial of labor, nor is six hours even though the patient may still be at 2 centimeters. Again, from the time contractions start until the patient enters the second stage of labor can be 20 hours or longer. The patient, who can be in real pain even though her cervix is not dilating, is, of course, not happy to hear that she still has many hours to go and is likely to give her eager consent if the doctor mentions "c-section." That is why I feel quite strongly that in the case of a primary cesarean section, a second opinion should be requested, preferably from a perinatologist or the chairman of the obstetrics department or even the chief obstetrics resident—in any event, from someone not in the attending obstetrician's group. The consultant can review the monitoring strip, determine the intensity of the contractions, examine the patient, and confer with the obstetrician, ensuring that a cesarean section will be performed only if the objective evidence justifies it. But how many women are going to request a second opinion? Not too many, I fear. They do not want to go through more labor. They are looking for an out, and if the doctor offers them one, they are usually delighted to take it.

Indeed, the major reason for repeat cesarean sections is patient request. The patient says, "I went through all that labor before, Doc, and ended up with a c-section anyway, so this time why don't we just go in in the first place?" It is true that there are no guarantees; the patient may again go through a long labor and again end up needing a cesarean section. This possibility is particularly likely for women who receive epidural anesthesia too early in labor, cutting down on the force of the contractions so that a cesarean section becomes necessary. When they become pregnant again, they have the same mindset about avoiding pain and their first question is: "I have an option, don't I? When can we schedule a c-section?" Insurance companies are protesting: "We're going to force these women to have VBACs. We can't have all these repeat sections." This is totally inappropriate; it is not their call. But women do need to be educated to the fact that cesarean sections are not without risk and should be performed only when the indications for them are very clear.

That said, I must admit that a cesarean section is exquisitely kind to the fetus. There is no battering of the head against the bones of the mother's pelvis. Cesarean section babies have nice round little heads, while vaginally delivered babies tend to look like coneheads. The only time this is not true is if the cesarean has followed a long trial of labor. If the baby has not been able to fit through the mother's pelvis, often its head becomes wedged, in which case another attendant in the operating room must go in underneath the sterile drapes, put a hand in the vagina, and dislodge the head, freeing the baby so that the obstetrician can lift it out.

VAGINAL BIRTH AFTER CESAREAN (VBAC)

In 1970 the rate for vaginal delivery after the woman had had a cesarean section to deliver a previous baby was 2.2 per 100 deliveries. In 1993 it was 25.4 per 100 deliveries. In general, the philosophy used to be "Once a section, always a section," but that began to change after obstetricians were allowed to perform abdominal surgery. When I was in training, obstetricians were very good at vaginal techniques, such as forceps delivery or even a vaginal hysterectomy, but they were not permitted to operate on the abdomen. A surgeon was called in to deliver a baby in distress or a mother in prolonged labor, and the procedure was simply to bivalve the uterus like a clam, to cut right down the middle. When the mother became pregnant again, that area of weakness, that suture line, was exactly where the uterine contractions to push the baby out also were, and with the onset of labor, it was conceivable that the uterus could rupture. Because sometimes the uterus ruptured even before the onset of active labor, the mother was almost always scheduled for a cesarean section at about 39 weeks, before she could go into labor. But then we obstetricians came into the surgical arena. Because we were inclined to think of the uterus as a muscle rather than an organ, we established that there is a noncontractile part of the uterus in the lower segment. With a transverse cut in this lower area instead of a vertical bivalving, the incision came in an area that does not contract during labor. Thus, women who had had a cesarean could later deliver vaginally without running too great a risk of the uterus rupturing.

This is only the case, however, if the cesarean was done for a nonrepetitive reason. To define repetitive: If a woman's first baby weighed 8 pounds and a cesarean section was done because her pelvis was too small to accommodate that size baby, that reason will hold true in every subsequent pregnancy as well because each succeeding baby is usually larger than the one before. With the first baby at 8 pounds, the next is most likely to be, say, 8.4 pounds, and the one after that 8.6 pounds. If the mother's pelvis was too small for the first baby, it is going to be too small for all the following babies. However, if her first cesarean was because of a breech presentation or because the mother was bleeding or for toxemia, and the cause does not reappear in a subsequent pregnancy, it is safe for her to attempt a vaginal delivery.

DELIVERY OF PREMATURE BABIES

In 1973 we did not perform a cesarean section if we believed the baby weighed less than five pounds. Even if we knew that the fetus was in distress, we waited and allowed it to be delivered vaginally because we did not have the means to keep a baby smaller than five pounds alive. The consequence was either a very ill or dead baby. In the 25 years since then, however, neonatal medicine and neonatal intensive care units have come into being, and if there is a compelling reason to do so, we now deliver the baby as early as 25 or 26 weeks.

At that age, at least twelve weeks short of full term, the average human fetus weighs one pound, nine ounces. The little mouse that comes out is not a pretty sight, not like a Gerber baby. It is tiny and scrawny and has very, very thin skin with little or no "baby fat" because fat is not deposited until the end of the pregnancy; the last couple of weeks of gestation are when babies plump up like ballpark franks. The ability of neonatalogists to keep such a tentative creature alive is impressive, with the determining factor being whether the baby can get past the breathing problems associated with the immaturity of the lungs. If the lungs are structurally functional, the baby will live, although there may be consequent neurological problems such as cerebral palsy or ocular problems such as retinopathies leading to blindness.

Fetal distress is a prime reason for a cesarean section at 26 weeks. Another is if the mother has toxemia, or preeclampsia, which can lead to convulsions and death. Knowing that the preeclamptic mother has a high risk of dying if the pregnancy continues, while delivery will bring about immediate improvement in her physical state, we go in and take the baby.

If the mother's life is in jeopardy from whatever cause, and if after considerable consultation and discussion we feel that delivering the baby will improve her status, we will deliver the baby even if it is previable. If the gestation is at 19 weeks, for instance, and the mother has invasive cancer, the mother's life has priority. If she is at 24 or 25 weeks, we ask the oncologists, "Can you wait two weeks? If we have just two more weeks, we know the baby is salvageable." If the answer is, "No, because our studies have shown that the mothers are going to die if they don't have this right now," then we have no choice but to deliver the baby. But such instances are very infrequent.

When the baby must be delivered early, whether we induce labor or do a cesarean depends on the position of the baby. If the baby's head is coming first, we will induce labor, but if it is a breech presentation, that is, the feet or buttocks are coming first, we do not allow the mother to deliver vaginally. When the baby is so small, the head is disproportionately large in relation to the rest of the body. A little butt comes out, but then the cervix closes around the head of the baby, entrapping it, and delivery of the rest of the baby becomes impossible.

When you have to deliver one of these premature babies weighing only a pound and some ounces, you hope it will be a girl, not for a sexist reason but because girl babies do better than boy babies. According to the statistics, 106 males are born for every 100 females. But at the end of a year, the ratio evens out, indicating that there is a higher neonatal death rate for males.

AGE OF THE FETUS

When we speak of a 26-week fetus, how is that age determined? Somewhat by ultrasound, which gives a picture of the baby's stage of development, but mostly by counting from the first day of the mother's last menstrual period. Conception may have occurred a couple of weeks later, but since there is seldom a way of knowing just when because intercourse may have occurred many times during the month, obstetricians go back to evidence the patient can attest to, the first day of her last menstrual period—another reason why it is important to keep a menstrual calendar. The counting is done from the first day rather than the last because some periods are five days, some are two, some are seven, but the first day is the first day.

The patient may say she is less than five weeks pregnant, and I ask, "What was the first day of your last menstrual period?"

"It was February 1st, and I was supposed to get my period March 1st but now it's March 20th." This makes her seven weeks pregnant. "No," she says. "The only time I had sex was February 15th. I am four and a half weeks pregnant."

However, obstetricians do not count like that. Clinically, she is seven weeks pregnant. In all obstetrical data, all the literature, all investigations, when gestational age is mentioned, it is based on the first day of the last menstrual period. Whether the fetus is 22 weeks or 26 or 28 is extremely important because at 22 weeks, it is not a viable baby; at 25 weeks, it may be; at 28 weeks, it almost certainly is.

POINTS TO REMEMBER

- In 1970 in the United States, one baby in 20 was delivered by cesarean section; in 1990, one baby in four was.
- Electronic monitoring is indispensable for checking the status of the baby and the effectiveness of labor.
- The average length of the first stage of labor is 20 hours for a first-time mother.
- All possibility of a natural birth should be exhausted before a cesarean section is resorted to.
- Risk of hemorrhage or infection is eight to ten times greater with a cesarean section than with vaginal birth.
- A fetal heartbeat going below 100 beats a minute or above 160 is an indication of fetal distress.
- A woman who has had a cesarean for a reason other than that the baby is too large can often deliver vaginally subsequently.
- Babies can be delivered as early as 26 weeks' gestation and survive.
- If the mother's life is in danger but the fetus is previable, the mother's life takes precedence. If the fetus is at 26 weeks or beyond, every effort is made to save both.

13

THE DARK SIDE OF OBSTETRICS

∾

MATERNAL MORBIDITY AND MORTALITY • TOXEMIA OF
PREGNANCY • DELIVERY OF THE BABY • AMNIOTIC FLUID
EMBOLISM • UTERINE ATONY • PLACENTA ACCRETA •
INFANT MORBIDITY AND MORTALITY • BREECH BIRTH •
SHOULDER DYSTOCIA • SIZE OF THE BABY • HERMAPH-
RODITISM • SEX AND WEIGHT • CONGENITAL DEFECTS •
THE FOUR STAGES OF OBSTETRICS •

Without in any way wishing to encourage pessimism, I would be
happier if parents went into the delivery room with some of the same
trepidation they experience when one of them is going into surgery,
or even taking an airplane. The surgery or the flight in all likelihood
will be successful, but people have a heightened concern; they sort of
hold their breath until it is over. Not so when they go into labor and
delivery. They expect everything to be fine, they assume they are
guaranteed a happy ending, but, as the song says, "It ain't necessarily
so." Much can happen, and that is why obstetricians are highly
trained, so that they can deal with the unexpected, with emergencies.

MATERNAL MORBIDITY AND MORTALITY

There is no happier time than the birth of a baby, but pregnancy and
childbirth are not without risk. As the tombstones in colonial ceme-
teries attest, early American settlers tried valiantly to fulfill the Biblical command to be fruitful and multiply, but to do so, many a
husband had to take a succession of wives as one after another died in
childbirth. The phrase, "She died in childbirth," remained current
until recent times. In 1872 one in every ten women in the United
States died in childbirth, and as late as 1915 the number of women,

especially nonwhite women, dying as a result of pregnancy and its complications was 1500 for every 100,000 live births.

Although the maternal mortality rate in the United States today is down to 7.4 deaths per 100,000 live births, pregnancy and childbirth remain the eleventh leading cause of death in women of childbearing age. Even in this technologically advanced era, we need to maintain a healthy respect for the complications that can lie just around the corner in any pregnancy and delivery.

Preeclampsia, hemorrhage, and infection used to be the most common causes of maternal mortality, but today death from thromboembolic disease—dislodged blood clots—leads the way. Hemorrhage occurs most often with ectopic pregnancies in the first trimester, with placenta previa in the third trimester, and with placenta accreta at the time of delivery. Death due to infection is less common today because of the availability of antibiotics, but women who have a cesarean section are at significantly increased risk of developing an infection over women giving birth vaginally, which is why, as noted, the obstetrician waits for every possibility of a vaginal birth to be exhausted before moving to a cesarean section.

Toxemia of Pregnancy. *Preeclampsia, pregnancy-induced hypertension*, and *toxemia* are three names for the same thing, an insidious process that is little understood, occurs after 20 weeks of pregnancy, and can be deadly. Three factors define toxemia in the pregnant woman: protein in the urine; high blood pressure; and swelling, or edema. Unfortunately, these are three things that the woman does not know she has unless or until she goes for prenatal checkups.

Women tend to say, "All I do is pee in a cup, the nurse takes my blood pressure, the doctor measures my tummy, and I'm out of there. I'm paying all this money just for that?" Right, because if the little cup of urine shows 4+ protein, and your blood pressure has gone from 110 over 70 to 150 over 95, and you can no longer wear your wedding ring because your fingers are swollen, you have preeclampsia without knowing it. And if you do not take care of it, it is like the Terminator: It destroys. There is a 30 percent probability of loss of the baby, 10 to 15 percent probability that the mother will die if preeclampsia progresses to eclampsia (convulsions). The toxemia of pregnancy accounts for many of the deaths of pregnant women in underdeveloped countries where there are not doctors doing that trivial thing of checking the urine and taking the blood pressure.

On the portico at Lying-In Hospital in Chicago, a series of shields are inscribed with the names of the greats in obstetrics, but one shield is blank. It is awaiting the name of the person who discovers the etiology of toxemia. Why does it happen? What causes it? We do not know. All we know is that first-time mothers are at higher risk of developing it, as are African-American mothers, patients in the lower socioeconomic classes, patients who do not receive prenatal care, overweight women, and women with diabetes.

Residents in training are alert to the slightest signs of toxemia, but when obstetricians go out into private practice, they tend to forget about the possibility. I have been called in many times and asked, "Dr. Thornton, what do you think is wrong here?"

"Tell me the history."

"Well, her blood pressure was 100 over 70 when she was seven weeks, and now it's 140 over 85, not that high."

"What's the urine like?"

"She's only spilling one- or two-plus protein."

"How much weight has she gained?"

"Eight pounds in a month."

Because the doctor knows that heavier women tend to have higher blood pressure and because the patient has only a slight amount of protein in her urine, he has dismissed the signs and told the patient to go home and stay in bed, and now he is wondering why she and the baby are doing poorly. But (as outlined in chapter 5) weight gain during pregnancy should be no more than two pounds in the first trimester, and from then until delivery, three-fourths to one pound a week, which adds up to three or four pounds a month. If the woman has gained five pounds in a week, that may be one of the signs of developing toxemia; she does not yet have it, but it is a red flag. Add in that her blood pressure is a little high, and that is two out of three of the signs; and normal pregnant women do not "spill" protein in their urine. That is three out of three signs, and I am wondering why her doctor is even consulting me. It is as obvious as can be that the woman is preeclamptic. The treatment? Delivery. There is no other. The toxemia cannot be allowed to go on because it can kill the mother and kill the baby, while, with delivery of the baby, it most often is resolved within a few days.

Delivery of the Baby. When preeclampsia is detected at 26 weeks, is immediate delivery indicated or do you wait and try to gain more time for the fetus to develop? There are no definitive guidelines, so common sense comes into play. If the hospital has a good neonatal intensive care unit, the likelihood of the baby's surviving—even though, at 26 weeks, it weighs only a pound and a half—is good, and it protects the mother's life if the baby is delivered. It is when the baby is previable that you are desperate to gain more time. Usually the preeclampsia occurs after 20 weeks, and the baby is viable at 26 weeks. Between weeks 20 and 26, what do you do? You keep the mother in the hospital, administer magnesium sulfate to head off convulsions, and keep a constant check on her liver enzymes and her uric acid, hoping against hope to stave off full-blown eclampsia. If you cannot, then you have to save the mother. If you can, then you deliver the baby at 26 weeks because studies have shown there is no advantage to keeping it there longer. The vessels carrying oxygen to the baby are constricted, inhibiting its growth, and even if the pregnancy were to go to 33 weeks the baby would probably remain at 26-week size.

In delivering the preeclamptic patient, we give her magnesium sulfate to reduce the likelihood of seizures and Pitocin to send her into labor. Or we go immediately to a cesarean section if her blood pressure is 210 over 100, for example, if she is spilling protein, has visual disturbances and a severe headache, and if she has abdominal pain. These are the signs of severe preeclampsia. The patient is not putting out any urine, her kidneys have shut down, and the capsule around her liver is starting to rupture. The bottom can fall out very fast with a patient who only a short time before was saying, "I don't feel anything. Everything is fine."

My professors claimed that there should no longer be any eclampsia because obstetricians should detect preeclampsia and prevent it from progressing into convulsions. If a woman does have seizures, they said, either she has had no access to health care or somebody has missed the boat.

One way of missing the boat is forgetting that many young women normally have a blood pressure of 90 over 60 or 70 over 40, which is very low. If their blood pressure then goes to 120 over 80, which in another person would be normal, they may have the beginnings of preeclampsia. Any 30 point increase in the systolic or 15 point increase in the diastolic is high blood pressure and is important. What matters is not the absolute figures but the change, and that is what a doctor should be picking up.

When I was in the navy and stationed at Bethesda, I was sent to Parris Island to help out. It was the rule there that a pregnant woman who came to the emergency room could not be sent home until her case was presented to an obstetrician. One night I got a call at two a.m. from a nonchalant emergency room resident who said, "Hey, Doc, we got a patient here, she's about 34 weeks and she's complaining of persistent indigestion, heartburn."

I asked, "What's her blood pressure?"

"It's not that high—130 over 84."

"Did you take her urine?"

"It's just one or two plus."

"Admit her," I ordered.

"What! Why can't I just send her home with some antacids?" She was fine, he thought. A little bit of heartburn; blood pressure 130 over 80, not a big deal; a little protein, which could be a contaminant from a vaginal discharge. Why was I saying, "Get her into Labor and Delivery right now"? I must be out of my mind.

But we had no sooner gotten the patient into the labor room than she had an eclamptic seizure and almost bit off her tongue. It was a mess, but finally we got her controlled and delivered the baby. When it was over, the emergency room guy looked at me wonderingly. "How did you know? How did you know?"

"It was the heartburn," I told him. "With that kind of pain in that part of the abdomen, it can mean that the capsule of the liver is rupturing." That is the insidiousness of this illness. As seemingly innocuous a thing as heartburn, if it goes hand in hand with elevated blood pressure and protein in the urine, warns that eclampsia is just around the corner.

Preeclampsia is relentless once it starts. The blood pressure can go down for one or two readings but when it comes back up, it is higher than ever. Many a doctor has been fooled by a return of the blood pressure to a normal reading of 100 over 70. When it becomes elevated again, the doctor goes into denial: "It cannot be preeclampsia. Let's bring in the neurologist because the patient has visual disturbances. Let's bring in the renal specialist because she is not urinating. Let's bring in the hypertension specialist to give her medication for the blood pressure." Pretty soon there is a doctor there for the eyes, for the kidneys, for the weight gain, for the blood pressure, and they are ordering CAT scans and every kind of medication. Then the perinatalogist walks in and says, "She doesn't need any of those things. She needs to be delivered."

Let me make one further point before leaving the subject of preeclampsia. While swelling of the hands and feet can be a sign of preeclampsia, swelling of the feet alone, without high blood pressure and without protein in the urine, is considered to be a good sign. Why this should be so, I do not know, but it has long been observed that a little bit of fluid in a pregnant woman's ankles in the last trimester is associated with a good outcome. Conversely, little or no fluid in the ankles is a cause for concern.

This does not mean that a woman who has had two children can say, with her third pregnancy, "Oh, my ankles always swell up," and let it go at that. She may, without her knowledge, be spilling protein, and she can end up in dire straits if she is not being checked by someone who can ask the right questions in order to arrive at the right diagnosis.

Amniotic Fluid Embolism. Amniotic fluid embolism, which is very rare, is caused by the injudicious use of Pitocin. Pitocin pumps need to be carefully monitored to allow for a relaxation period between uterine contractions. If the uterus is not allowed to rest, titanic contractions push amniotic fluid into the maternal veins, and the particulate matter in the fluid goes to the mother's lungs, where it acts as an anticoagulant, causing hemorrhaging and leading to the mother's death within minutes.

Even without Pitocin, contractions may begin to come too fast. If we see on the monitor a line that stays high instead of going up and down like camel humps, we try to get the mother to relax and per-haps give her a medication to slow the contractions. The patient may be okay, but we want to avoid any risk of an amniotic fluid embolism because the mortality rate is as high at 95 percent.

A vivid case of amniotic fluid embolism happened when I was a resident observing the forceps delivery of the baby of a 19-year-old patient. We were concerned about the baby, which had an Apgar score of one at one minute, and were working to resuscitate it when the mother said, "I can't breathe." The nurse anesthetist was right there and gave her oxygen. The patient was fighting the mask, and then . . . nothing. There was no heart rate. "Code, Labor and Delivery Room!" People ran, incredulous that they were going to Labor and Delivery for a Code for cardiac arrest because it virtually never happens in that part of the hospital. When the emergency team got there, we were pumping on her chest and beating her. They took over, and while they were working on the patient, I remembered a recommendation I had read to draw a sample of blood, tape the tube of blood to the wall, and keep looking at it. Normal blood will clot quite rapidly and you will see the serum separating. But this patient's blood did not clot, and suddenly she was bleeding from her nose and ears and IV site and just everywhere. In minutes she had bled to death. It was like witnessing an airplane crash. Everyone in the room was crying because it was so unexpected, such a shock.

I was present at the autopsy, and absolutely nothing was visible to account for the tragedy. Not until weeks later when the reports came back from the laboratory did we learn that the cause of death was amniotic fluid that had entered the patient's bloodstream, disabling the clotting mechanism.

This was my first maternal death, and doubly overwhelming because the patient was so young. It happened when monitors were just being introduced and it was not routine to insert them. A monitor would have given us warning that the contractions were coming too fast or not coming down to a relaxing baseline; after that the hospital made them mandatory for every obstetric patient.

Uterine Atony. Women who have had five or more children—grand multiparas, they are called—are at increased risk for uterine atony, the failure of the uterus to clamp down and control excessive postpartum bleeding. Like a much-worn girdle, the uterus may have lost its elasticity and not snap back like it used to. An obstetrician who is delivering a grand multipara anticipates this possibility and arranges for the typing and cross-matching of four units of blood ahead of time so that it is at hand in the event of postpartum hemorrhage.

Uterine atony can also be a consequence of a baby with shoulder dystocia (discussed later). The uterus been contracting and contracting and contracting in an attempt to eject the baby, and sometimes it becomes exhausted, too exhausted to keep on contracting in order to return to its firm involuted state. In such instances, Pitocin is given to induce contractions. Massage is stepped up. The blood bank is alerted. Transfusions are started. If despite all measures the bleeding continues, the race to the operating room is on. Hysterectomy is the only recourse at such a time.

Placenta Accreta. After a vaginal delivery, if the placenta has not come out within 30 minutes, placenta accreta becomes a possibility. Placenta accreta occurs when, at the beginning of the pregnancy, unbeknownst to anyone, the placenta attaches itself directly to the wall of muscle of the uterus rather than on a filmy thin layer (Nitabuch's layer) that sheds after delivery. If the placenta penetrates *into* the uterine muscle, the condition is called placenta increta. The most extreme and dangerous type of placenta accreta is placenta percreta, a condition in which the placenta penetrates through the full thickness of the uterus and may invade adjacent structures such as the bladder. Placenta percreta carries a 10 percent risk of maternal death.

In a delivery, after the baby has arrived, all the excitement seems to be over and I as the obstetrician sit and wait for the placenta to be delivered. And sometimes I wait and wait. The father has gone with the baby to the nursery, and the mother and I are there but nothing is happening. I wonder if perhaps the placenta is just lazy, which is what I am praying is the case when I gingerly go into the uterus and probe for a cleavage plane. If there is a cleavage plane, the placenta separates from the wall and comes out. If not, if only stringy pieces of placenta can be dragged out, big trouble lies ahead. The uterus is not going to contract because it is not empty; the villi, the fingerlike projections of the placenta, are still in there; and the uterus continues to bleed at the rate of a pint of blood per minute because there are still open channels and the intervillous spaces are big spaces.

In the worst scenario, you massage the uterus and the patient keeps bleeding. You give her methergine and the bleeding goes on. You inject prostaglandin directly into the uterine muscle and still the blood comes. The uterus may become a little firm, but then it grows boggy again. The bleeding goes on. Now you have to act quickly and systematically, without hesitation, in order to save a life. You have to prepare for surgery, either to tie off the major vessels that supply blood to the uterus or to do an emergency hysterectomy.

A patient told me, "You're always so calm in front of your patients, Dr. Thornton, that I knew it was really serious when I heard you say, 'Goddamn it, I can't feel a pulse!'" And it was serious. She had no blood pressure, and the amount of blood coming out was unbelievable. We were transfusing her, but her blood volume was down to almost nothing. I had to operate extremely rapidly, in a postpartum patient's anatomy that is not the same as in a nonpregnant lady and with all the difficulty of working with spongy, soft tissues and blood vessels so mushy that clamps will scarcely hold. Not easy, but fortunately the patient pulled through and is fine now.

The woman who has been through this knows that it was a life-threatening situation and you had to remove her uterus to prevent her bleeding to death, but times goes by and someone makes the off-hand comment, "Oh, you had a hysterectomy, you're not a woman anymore," and someone else suggests, "Why don't you sue?" "No . . . no . . . no," says the patient, but more months go by, the patient forgets it was an emergency, and the doctor is served with papers. Even though the doctor wins the suit, some very, very good physicians have given up the practice of obstetrics for just this reason.

INFANT MORBIDITY AND MORTALITY

Breech Birth. Not all babies arrive head first. In three percent of full-term births the presenting portion of the baby is the buttocks. If it is known in advance that it will be a breech birth in a first-time mother, a cesarean section is done, but sometimes the first clue comes when you examine the mother and see meconium on your fingers, at which point you ask yourself whether the baby is in distress or is something else happening. You test with your fingers, and if what you feel is not a hard head but the cheeks of the buttocks, you know this is a frank breech: The baby is folded like a safety pin, with the buttocks presenting first in the birth canal. Or you may feel feet, in which case it is a footling breech: The baby is sitting cross-legged like a Native American. Or one or both feet are through the cervix, and the baby is in what in diving is called a pike position. This is the worst of the positions because the umbilical cord can slip past the feet, be compressed by the cervix, and cause a lot of problems. Indeed, take any problem that can occur with a vaginal vertex (head-first) delivery, crank it up one hundred times, and that is what can go wrong in a breech delivery.

If it is a first baby, a cesarean section is recommended because the mother's pelvis has not been tested. But if this is the mother's second or third baby and the baby seems to be no larger than her first one, the physician may opt for a vaginal delivery. An assisted breech delivery is attempted when a patient has a frank breech, has had a good labor pattern, and has gone through the Friedman curve (see chapter 11)—two, four, six, eight centimeters—and easily becomes fully dilated.

Breech delivery is rapidly becoming a lost art, so when one is underway, the staff—medical students, residents, and pediatricians alike—usually crowd into the delivery room to watch. The baby's buttocks come out, and you as the obstetrician do not pull. You gently wrap a warm towel around the baby's buttocks—warm because you don't want to startle the baby so that it gasps while still inside the uterus and inhales meconium. With the towel in place, you do a Pinard maneuver to get the feet out: You go up behind the baby's thigh; put one finger in back of the knee and one in front; bend the knee so that the leg is doubled over and bring it out. Then you do the same thing to the other leg. Now both legs and the butt are hanging out of the vagina, and if someone happens to come into the delivery room at that moment, it can look frightening.

Next you loosen up the umbilical cord to make sure that it is neither entrapped nor compressed; if you feel pulsations in it, you know it is okay. Then you allow the mother's contractions to move the baby on down. However, the arms may now be above the baby's head, and when you go in to try to get an arm, all you feel is an armpit, in which case you go up the baby's back and sweep one of the arms across the chest and it comes down, then sweep the other across and it comes down. That is, the arms come down unless they are around the neck in what is called a supernuchal hitch. If this is the case, you have to know how to rotate the baby so that gravity brings the arms down.

Now that everything has been delivered except the head, you do the Mauriceau-Smellie-Veit maneuver, so-called after three of the greats in the early days of obstetrics. Hopefully, the cervix is still dilated. You put two of your fingers on the baby's lower jaw and your pinkie and thumb on the baby's cheekbones, slide your other hand up the back of the baby's head, push on its chin, and roll the baby out.

What if the cervix has not remained dilated but instead has clamped down around the baby's neck? You have all the rest of the baby out, but the head is still in there. When this happens, you pray and you ask for halothane, an anesthetic that produces uterine relaxation. This possible need for halothane is why, when you are going for a breech delivery, the patient needs to be set up for general anesthesia. With the cervix clamped down on the baby's head, you have to move really fast. You ask the anesthesiologist in a calm tone, "Can you give her some general anesthetic?" He or she knows the baby's head is trapped and administers halothane immediately.

With halothane, with luck, the uterus will relax and you can do the Mauriceau-Smellie-Veit maneuver to get the baby out of there. But if the uterus does not relax, then you need to do Duhrssen's incisions, which means making cuts in the cervix. Think about the situation: The baby's back and shoulders are out, the cervix is above them, and the head is trapped above the cervix. You have to take a pair of scissors and go in and try to cut the sides of the cervix. Often you cut more than you would have liked to and the incision extends up into the uterus, which starts bleeding heavily because that is where the arteries are that feed the cervix.

A calm head is the most important instrument an obstetrician can have. You say to yourself, "Okay, this has happened, this is what I am dealing with, I am doing the best I can, and I know I'll be in court three months from now." Most doctors do not want to go through that, so breech deliveries are becoming rare, the skill to do them is lost, and cesarean sections are commonplace. You can deliver a beautiful breech—beautiful because it is the baby's bottom rather than head that is getting the battering—and still be sued for malpractice because the baby turns out to have a learning disability and the parents blame it on the breech birth even though the breech delivery has had nothing to do with it.

Shoulder Dystocia. In a vaginal vertex birth, after the head has been delivered, the shoulders almost always follow promptly. But sometimes there comes the obstetrician's nightmare: shoulder dystocia, in which the baby's shoulders have become wedged behind the mother's pelvis. There is no predicting it. Suddenly it is obvious that the baby is caught, and it is as though the ground opens up and plunges you into an abyss because it is so unexpected. The shoulders are not emerging; they are stuck, and the baby's head is turning blue and its eyes are looking at you. Shoulder dystocia does not happen often, thank God, but when you are in the midst of it, you are fighting for the baby's life.

The Zavanelli maneuver, rarely performed, was successfully done on the television program *ER*, so millions of people now believe it is feasible to push the baby's head back in and then do a cesarean section. Maybe, but it is not easy. Everything is so tight that it is extremely difficult to get your hand in to push on the baby and try to reverse the cardinal movements of delivery. Furthermore, the baby has a compressible neck, and while you are pushing, the neck compresses but the head does not move. You do not have time to wait and see if keeping up the pressure will budge the baby. You only have a second or two; then you have to move on to the next thing to try.

You call for somebody to help because you need to have another person press hard on the mother's pubic bone to try to dislodge the shoulders while you attempt to maneuver the baby's head. Husbands are not useful at such a time. They are saying, "What's the matter? What's the matter?" We answer, "No problem," even though the rest of us know that it is a state of emergency. The nurse smiles at the father while she pushes down on the pubic bone, and you smile at him while you are pulling on the baby's head.

You dare not pull too hard for fear of causing Erb's palsy, a consequence of stretching the nerves that innervate the shoulder, making the baby's arm limp after you finally deliver it. You try hard not to have that happen, but sometimes you are stacking Erb's palsy up against a live baby, and you want a live baby at all costs.

You have placed the mother's knees way back, back toward her ears, to decrease the length of the vagina. The nurse is pushing down on the pubic bone. You are trying to corkscrew the baby back and forth to dislodge it. Meanwhile, you have to extend the episiotomy that you did earlier to get the head out. You go down on your knees to find where the episiotomy is, and you cut into the rectum. You have no choice. With luck, that will give you enough space to put your hand in and work the baby free. All this takes three or four minutes, not very long but they are the worst minutes of an obstetrician's life.

When you finally get the baby out, you look at it, praying that it does not have a flail arm because if it does, that arm will probably not function well for the rest of the baby's life, although sometimes Erb's palsy responds to therapy or spontaneously corrects itself.

Occasionally the recommendation is made to fracture the baby's clavicle if all else fails, but this does not take into account that the baby who gets stuck behind the pubic bone is likely to be chubby, not a skinny little thing, and the clavicle is cushioned. It would be like trying to fracture a bone through six inches of sponge, which is next to impossible. It sounds terrible that you would resort to breaking a baby's bone, but I would do it in a minute if I could; that is how desperate the situation is.

Not often but sometimes you pull and you pull and you pull, and finally you get the baby out but it is not breathing; it has been caught there too long. The Apgar score is zero over zero. The moment is devastating. I cannot begin to describe how awful it is. It was to be the happiest time: The show is starting, the curtain is rising on a life, the spotlight comes on, and . . . the baby is dead. You tried and you tried and you tried, but it was beyond human skill. The lactic acid buildup has exerted its effect on the baby's heart, the heart is not pumping anymore, and the baby is stillborn. You are the captain of the team so you are blamed, and you accept the blame because you understand the parents' grief and disappointment, but the truth is that you did everything you could.

Size of the Baby. The normal weight of the human baby is six to seven pounds, and the maternal pelvis is made for that size. Studies have shown that shoulder dystocia happens with large babies of nine or ten pounds, although it can also happen when the baby is eight pounds, or even seven pounds if the mother has a small pelvis. You do not know it is coming until it hits, which is one more reason why I am not a proponent of births outside of a hospital setting. Highly skilled people going into action in split seconds are needed if this mother and this baby, who have come so far together, are going to have the best possible shot at continuing on. The mother can help, too, by not gaining 60 pounds during her pregnancy, which results in larger babies.

Hermaphroditism. Occasionally, after an uneventful birth, you look at the baby and see that it has ambiguous genitalia. Girls have indoor plumbing, boys have outdoor plumbing, but with some babies you are not sure what the plumbing is: It looks like a penis, but it does not look like a penis. In such a situation, I was taught to tell the parents that they have a girl because, however much it pains me to say so, in our culture boys are more acceptable than girls, and if you announce it is a boy but it later turns out to be a girl, people may be disappointed. On the other hand, if you say it is a girl and it turns out to be a boy, they tend to be pleased. Because the sex of the baby is always the first question parents ask, you do have to say something without waiting for the results of chromosomal studies that will indicate which sex the baby really is.

Not being able to tell the baby's sex just by looking at it does not mean that the child will grow up to be homosexual or bisexual. But parents do not necessarily know that and they may unconsciously turn against the baby. It makes a difference how a baby is treated from the moment it is born, and if the parents' reaction is confused or unfavorable, it can have a lifelong impact on the patient's sense of identity, so I feel it is best to let some hours go by before the situation is discussed with the parents.

Sex and Weight. The first questions parents ask obstetricians are always: "Is it a boy or girl?" and "How much does it weigh?" What the parents should be asking is: Is the baby alive? Is it blue? Are the Apgar scores okay? Is the baby breathing on its own? The least important thing in the world at this juncture is how much the baby weighs, but when I say that I don't know, the parents look at me as though I have just failed an obstetrician's most important test. The fact is, there is no scale in the delivery room. There used to be, but if it differed from the one in the nursery, it could seem that the baby had lost four or five ounces when really the weight difference was due to a discrepancy in the scales. Many states, therefore, passed laws that the only scale should be in the nursery. There the baby is weighed every day, and if the scale registers a loss, it is a genuine loss, not a difference in calibration.

Congenital Defects. Even though the National Institutes of Health said in 1980 that ultrasound testing need not be done routinely, I, and every other obstetrician I know, feel that it is important to identify gross structural defects in the fetus prenatally. To that end, we do at least one ultrasound test during the pregnancy. There are, however, lesser abnormalities that either are not identifiable on ultrasound or not severe enough to justify termination of pregnancy, and these show up at delivery. Examples of such correctable anomalies are a cleft lip, an extra finger, or a little tail.

Again, out of compassion, nothing is said to the parents immediately after the baby is born. All the hours of labor have been a long haul, and you do not want to disturb the shining moment when the baby arrives. Hopefully, the head and cheeks are normal, and the swaddled baby can be shown to the parents without their needing to know about the tuft of hair growing in the back of the baby's behind or the imperforate anus or the extra toes. After the baby has been shown to the parents, we say, "We have to take the baby to the nursery because it looks a little chilled."

The neonatalogist and the pediatric neurologist and the pediatric cardiologist—whatever specialists are needed—descend on the nursery, and if decisions have to be made right away, they will confer with the father. If it is a cardiac defect, that is not usually known at birth because so many structures in the baby are changing and closing in the 24 hours after it is born. With the shortened hospital stays now in vogue, this can be a problem because mothers are not trained to look for duskiness, and if they do not recognize until two or three days later that something is wrong, it can be too late. In the old days, nurses who were skilled at recognizing problems would say, "That baby just doesn't look right," and specialists would arrive to examine the child. Now that we no longer have that safety net, it is important that a pediatrician give the baby a thorough examination before it leaves the hospital.

Any more detailed discussion of birth defects would take us beyond my area of expertise. I am an obstetrician, and if the defect does not appear on ultrasound but is only apparent at the birth of the baby, I hand the baby off to the pediatrician and he or she takes over responsibility at that point.

THE FOUR STAGES OF OBSTETRICS

The majority of fathers- and mothers-to-be know little or nothing about the dark side of obstetrics that we obstetricians deal with on a day-to-day basis. For them, everything is beautiful and they will be presented with a pink-cheeked, smiling baby, which is indeed the way it usually works out. Parents do not need to have the apprehensions about childbirth that were common in earlier centuries. The mind set for women then was, "I might not survive this," and many of them did not. Death in childbirth was an everyday occurrence, a fact of life. But no more.

The practice of obstetrics has gone through four stages. In the first stage, we concentrated on ensuring that the mother lived. Everything else was secondary. The next step was to make certain not only that she lived but that she was well, that she was discharged from the hospital without an infection, with a neatly repaired episi-otomy, and without a fistula. It was no good to pull her through childbirth only to have her have a fistula that resulted in her uri-nating or defecating through her vagina. After we got good at seeing that did not happen, we turned our attention to making certain we had live babies. And the fourth stage has been making sure that the babies are born healthy.

In the United States we have achieved these four goals, but in many countries obstetrics is still in the stage of "Let's hope we can get a live mother out of this," if indeed the mother is not still out in the countryside having her baby without help after three days of labor, and if she survives this ordeal, having fistula formation that later allows infection to kill her. I paint this picture only to make it clear why specialists in obstetrics are needed. It is not true that anyone can deliver a baby. If a taxicab driver delivers a baby, that baby was ready to arrive. The driver was not confronted with a foot hanging out of the vagina or the mother's hemorrhaging. These are emergencies that the movies do not show but that the obstetri-cian has to deal with, and deal with quickly and surely if it outcome is to be a live and healthy mother along with a live and healthy baby.

POINTS TO REMEMBER

- A happy ending is customary but not guaranteed in obstetrics, and some degree of concern is appropriate when a woman goes into the delivery room.
- Thromboembolic clots, toxemia, hemorrhage, and infection are the most common causes of maternal mortality.
- Toxemia in the pregnant woman is identified by three signs: protein in the urine, elevated blood pressure, and edema—signs that are detectable only by regular prenatal checkups.
- Most breech births are delivered by cesarean section.
- The baby's sex and weight are the least important questions to ask about a newborn; whether it is alive, and breathing nor-mally, with an adequate supply of oxygen in the blood, are the most important.

14

MIDWIVES AND BIRTHING CENTERS

❧

"Some of my best friends are . . ." Fill in the blank with any descriptive word, and what it usually means is that you do not socialize with or admire such persons but at the same time you do not wish to be seen as prejudiced. That being the case, I hope you will not assume I am being dismissive when I say that some of my best friends are midwives, but the fact is that I would not have the empathy I have with patients had I not trained in obstetrics in the midst of a good midwifery program at Roosevelt Hospital in New York City. I would have been like many of my colleagues in obstetrics who have the clinical, pathological, this-is-a-disease type of approach to a patient, looking at the monitor instead of the patient with an air of, "Okay, let's get this over with."

As a resident, my first exposure to, and experience with, women in labor had me dealing with them shoulder-to-shoulder with midwives. With all the tact in the world, the midwives would say, "Dr. Thornton, you don't really want to do that. Wouldn't it be better to . . . ? Don't you want to . . . ? Don't you suppose a warm blanket might feel good?" They were, in effect, saying, "Dr. Thornton, be human. Do the kind thing," as opposed to the doctors' approach: "How dilated is she? What we are going to do now is . . ."—the clinical world versus the human world of softness and gentleness. The latter are qualities obstetricians should have but that are hard for them to acquire unless they have trained with midwives.

The approach of midwives to childbirth is that it is a natural and wonderful experience to be shared by the mother and father and attendants. It is a sharing, that is, unless something goes wrong, at which point the midwife is yelling, "Get the doctor!" and the physician on duty is swearing because he or she has to come in and rescue the midwife. But even when I got to be chief resident and was the one who had to do the rescuing—dealing with forceps deliveries, breech deliveries, emergency cesarean sections, episiotomy breakdowns, and such things—I still remained grateful to the midwives for that early training in kindness. The only difference between us was that their training stopped there while mine went on.

This difference in training is why I believe that midwives should only practice in a hospital setting or in a doctor's practice, not in a private practice separate from a hospital. It is wonderful to have them there during the hours of labor, watching the monitors and ironing out the perineum. But for midwives to have a freestanding birthing center where certified nurse-midwives deliver the babies is not, I think, a good idea because of the possible eventualities described in chapter 13, "The Dark Side of Obstetrics." The monetary cost to the patient is less, but midwives do not have the advanced skills necessary to deal with emergency situations.

I expressed this opinion in the hearing of a midwife, and for the next year she did not speak to me at conferences or when we met on the labor and delivery floor. Then one evening just before midnight I got a call at home—a most reluctant call judging from the tone of voice; it was the midwife saying that her patient had been stuck at eight centimeters for three hours and needed a cesarean section. By rights, I should have dressed her down for not talking to me for a year and then expecting me to come out at that hour to help her out of a jam, but I did not. I went along to the hospital and was greeted by glares from the patient and her husband, who did not want anything to do with doctors.

I asked the midwife, "How are her contractions? If they're weak, we need to give her Pitocin. If they're strong, we need to do a c-section."

"She doesn't have an internal monitor," said the midwife. "I don't know how strong they are."

So I had to put in a monitor and wait two hours to determine the strength of the contractions, which did prove to be strong enough. That indicated the need for cesarean section. "Can't you wait a little longer?" the husband asked, obviously thinking that I had come in there like the hired gun with a scalpel and was going to do whatever I wanted to do. This kind of situation is why doctors do not like to cover midwives; it is not your patient, you have not developed a relationship with the patient and her husband that allows them to trust you, and if something goes wrong, which it usually has because otherwise you would not have been called in, you are the one who gets blown out of the water.

When I did the cesarean section, there was a substance similar to pea soup coming out of the lady's uterus, *thick* pea soup. I looked at the midwife. It was not fresh meconium; it was so old it was turning yellow. "Meconium," I warned the neonatologist standing by. I delivered the baby and suctioned its nose and mouth to get as much of the stuff out as possible, then handed it over to the neonatologist. An obstetrician's ears are always tuned to that first cry. I heard nothing. I looked at the midwife again.

"I didn't see any meconium when she was in labor," she insisted defensively. "There wasn't anything there."

The baby's Apgar scores were 1 and 4. My babies do not come out with Apgar scores of 1 and 4, I thought. Why am I in the midst of this? I took a sample of blood from the cord for an analysis of the blood gases, which tells how long the intrauterine hypoxia (low oxygen) has been going on and whether the baby has simply had the cord around its neck or something more long-range has been happening. The blood gases showed that this baby had been in trouble for a long time.

The midwife, who was at the mother's head, asked, "Dr. Thornton, how long will Mrs. X be in the hospital?" I did not answer because the mother had begun to bleed heavily from her uterus and I was saying to myself, "I just hope she gets off the table alive." The husband remarked, "You're kind of quiet down there, Dr. Thornton."

"I'm busy. I'll talk to you after I finish this." Because the baby had been wedged in for so many hours, there was a laceration in the mother's uterus that kept bleeding and bleeding. Over and over I said to the circulating nurse, "More sutures. Can I have more sutures, please?" I was throwing them in, trying to stop the hemorrhaging, and the neonatologist was struggling to suction meconium out of the baby's lungs and from under its larynx; all the while the midwife was fluttering around asking how long this was going to take, and if the father could go the nursery with the baby to take more pictures and find out the baby's weight.

Finally I got the bleeding stopped, but not before the lady had lost at least four pints of blood. "There was a little bit more bleeding than I would have liked," I told the mother euphemistically. "We're going to have to follow you to make sure you have the ability to make more red blood cells and to keep a watch out for infection. And the baby will be going to the neonatal intensive care section." And that was all I felt I could say to the parents. Anything more, any details about how nearly mother and baby had been lost, would only sound self-serving, and the answer would come back: "Oh, you big-time doctors, you only say that to run down midwives."

I do not run down midwives. They are wonderful women who taught me everything I know about being kind to patients. But when push comes to shove, as can happen in a split second in obstetrics, training—high-level, intensive medical training—is what matters, not that there is a nice person there to hold your hand. The nice person stroking your hand may have to sit by you and watch you die if there is not skilled medical help immediately available.

Free-standing birthing centers claim that they are safe because they only accept low-risk patients. However, 40 percent of high-risk patients come from the low-risk population, and in fact, almost 50 percent of the patients these centers handle have to be transferred to a hospital. With lay midwives instead of certified nurse-midwives, the record is worse. Lay midwives have had no standardized training, no certification. You might as well have your cousin deliver your baby. Indeed, if your cousin has seen a number of deliveries, she can call herself a lay midwife; there is nothing to stop her. Just the other day, a patient was literally dropped off on the front steps of our hospital. When she regained consciousness, she asked, "What happened? Why am I here? Where is the midwife?" Long gone, we told her, because you were hemorrhaging and she did not know what to do.

Giving birth should be simple, midwives say. Mother Nature knows what to do. Yes, but Mother Nature is not always predictable. She gives us sunshine and balmy breezes and gently lapping water, true, but she also gives us tornadoes and mudslides and hurricanes, and they can kill you. If a hurricane is coming, you do not say, "Let me go stand on the seawall and watch." You try to get to a protected place where you can ride out the storm safely. In obstetrics, that protected place is a hospital, so if your choice is to be attended by a midwife, choose one practicing in a birthing center within a hospital or no farther away than across the street and connected to the hospital by a stat corridor that zooms you through.

As I explained previously, *stat* is from the Latin *statim*, "immediately." And immediate is the response you want when there is a problem in obstetrics and not one but two lives are at stake.

POINT TO REMEMBER

- If you want a midwife to deliver your baby, choose one who practices within a hospital setting so that help is available in an emergency.

15

BREAST-FEEDING

❧

IMMUNE COMPETENCY • BONDING • WEANING •

The answer I give my patients when they ask about breast-feeding is: "Do you want me to say what I am supposed to tell you or what I really think?"

What I am supposed to tell you is that breast-feeding is marvelous, the natural way to nourish a child, desirable for the antibodies it passes along and because it promotes closeness and bonding. But what I would also like to tell a new mother is not to feel guilty if breast-feeding is not for you because you sense you would have a low tolerance for it, because you have other children at home, because you will be returning to work, or because you do not fancy whipping out a private part of your body in the midst of company or a church service to feed the baby. In deciding whether or not to breast-feed, you must first define what kind of person you are and the nature of your lifestyle and then make up your mind irrespective of the arguments of the La Leche League, which is a wonderful organization but, in my opinion, inclined to go too far in its proselytizing for breast-feeding.

I encourage my patients first to consider breast-feeding but then I add that they have an option, an option I chose for myself. I tell them that my two children were raised on Similac because I knew that after nine months of pregnancy and 23 hours of labor, my body was not up to breast-feeding and my demanding schedule would not permit it; and neither my bonding with them nor their health was in the least affected by their being bottle-fed. Often the patient's response is a big grin. "Dr. Thornton, I'm so happy you said that because I don't want to breast-feed but I've been afraid to admit it because I know you're supposed to do it."

There are women who just love to breast-feed and thrive on it, and for them the choice is easy. But some women have inverted nipples, some do not have enough breast tissue to breast-feed, and for some it is exceedingly painful. There is no guarantee that, however natural breast-feeding is, it will be an automatic success, as is evidenced by the calls I get from mothers with swollen breasts or cracked nipples or infections of the breast. More than 60 percent of women in the United States elect to breast-feed, but most mothers experience some difficulty with nursing and most do not continue nursing for as long as they had originally intended.

Breast-fed babies need feeding more often than bottle-fed babies—about every two hours versus every four hours. Among the breast-fed babies, mothers tell me, are three types. There is the prince or princess who turns its head away, communicating, "I don't want it now. I'll get it later." There is the thinker, the baby who cannot make up its mind whether or not it wishes to nurse. And then there is the barracuda who vigorously latches on to a breast and stays there seemingly forever. The books say "ten minutes on each breast," but in reality some babies take up to an hour or more. If the mother has other children to take care of, breast-feeding can take more time than she has to spend. If the mother has no time at all to spend because she works outside the home, she has to express the milk from her breasts, put it in a bottle, and have somebody take the bottle to the house to feed the baby. While I strongly believe that all *premature* infants should be breast-fed, I do believe that women with healthy, strong babies should be able to exercise their option not to breast-feed without being made to feel guilty and neglectful.

Companies promoting formula in third-world nations have come under fire in recent years and been compared to "drug lords," but I believe the comparison is too harsh because the indictment does not take into account the fact that in underdeveloped countries women have babies so close together that they do not have time to breast-feed one baby sufficiently well before another arrives. This is why there is so much malnutrition among infants and a high prevalence of maternal depletion syndrome, a situation that the use of formula can remedy.

IMMUNE COMPETENCY

Breast milk provides a specific antibody (IgA) to the newborn, as well as some lymphoctyes, which are immunologically important cells.

But, in fact, babies are born immune-competent. While they receive additional antibodies from the breast milk, all the time they are developing their own, and bottle-fed babies are no more prone to infection than breast-fed ones.

BONDING

Feeding the baby is unquestionably a time of closeness between mother and baby, but as far as my observation goes, it makes not the slightest bit of difference whether the baby has a part of mother in its mouth or the nipple on a bottle. Whether it is breast or bottle, it is the interaction between mother and baby that counts—the coos, soft words, and touching.

WEANING

To turn off the tap, you have to trick your body by wearing a tight binder. The bra you wore before you became pregnant makes a perfectly good breast binder because it is now too small. You wear it all the time, taking an analgesic such as Motrin or aspirin or Tylenol for the pain. When you take a shower, turn your back to the shower head because the impact of the water stimulates the nipples and causes milk production. For the same reason, your husband must not touch your nipples. If the breasts are warm or engorged, ice packs help. Crush some ice cubes and put the slush in a Ziplock bag and slip it inside your bra. After awhile the breasts will catch on to the fact that there is nothing happening and will cease milk production.

As a female obstetrician, I often hear from a patient, "What would you do if you were me, Dr. Thornton? My sister's breast-feeding and my mother tells me I ought to, but I have my doubts about it."

"I'm not you," I reply. "But after you have weighed the pros and cons of breast-feeding, if you decide to bottle-feed your baby, go ahead and don't feel any compunction about it. Believe me, you'll have plenty of other opportunities to feel guilty in relation to your child before you're through. Don't get hung up on this one."

In sum, I think a woman should do as she likes. Some women

want the experience. Some say it does not make a great deal of difference to them one way or the other so they will give breast-feeding a try for a few weeks or months. And some say, "I shudder at the thought of exposing my breasts and having the baby chewing on my body for three months." Each of these three reactions is understandable. It really is the woman's choice.

POINTS TO REMEMBER

- A baby is born immune-competent, and thus it is not imperative that he or she have mother's milk to remain healthy.
- Unless a baby is premature, the decision whether or not to breast-feed is really contingent on lifestyle and personal preference.

IV

FEMALE TROUBLE

❧

16

"FIBROIDS" OR MYOMAS

❦

CHARACTERISTICS AND TREATMENT

First, let's clear up a confusion of terms. The word *fibroid* is a misnomer. Tumors of the uterus arising within its smooth muscle are properly known as myomas—*myo-* being a combining form meaning "muscle." The word *fibroid* bears no relationship to uterine muscle; like the new word *factoid*, it has simply sneaked into our vocabulary, perhaps because it is easier to pronounce than *myoma*. My former chairman of OB/GYN would scream and hiss at anyone who was so misguided as to refer to a myoma as a fibroid. Since I am inclined to do the same, the proper term will be used throughout this chapter.

Myomas come in all sizes and look and feel hard and rubbery. In surgery, they appear as white balls, with a whorled appearance inside when cut. This has led to their being referred to casually as "fireballs of the uterus" even though they are not incendiary by any stretch of the imagination.

Myomas, which are rather like the eyes on a potato, are slow-growing and occur without any particular rhyme or reason. Twenty-five percent of all women have myomas, with the frequency rising to 50 percent in black women. This does not mean that 25 to 50 percent of women will need surgery, however, because for the most part myomas mind their own business. They can number from one to more than 50 in a uterus, and be the size of a pea—or even smaller, a pinhead—or, at the other extreme, grow as large as a cantaloupe, distorting the woman's abdomen.

Because there is so much variation, a woman who is told she has a myoma should ask a number of questions: Is it big? Is it single? Where is it located? Is it causing symptoms? Can you tell me more about it? She should not accept, "Fibroids—we've got to do a hysterectomy," as the last word. Myomas are the most frequent diagnosis leading to a hysterectomy, but an operation may or may not be the best way to handle the situation.

Myomas are estrogen-dependent for the most part; and as long as the ovaries are pushing out estrogen, myomas will continue to proliferate and/or grow. But at menopause, when there is not that estrogen output, they shrink. They do not entirely disappear but they will not be the same size when the woman is 60 as when she was 30. Therefore, a familiar refrain of doctors is: "Well, you know, menopause is coming and the myoma hasn't grown for a period of time. Why don't we just wait and see if it shrinks?"

Usually the myomas do shrink and there is no reason to be concerned about them anymore. However, if they are causing symptoms like irregular heavy bleeding or frequency of urination, that is another matter, as is the pressure of a myoma against the colon and the rectum leading to difficulty in defecation. Furthermore, it can be hard to distinguish between an ovarian cyst or tumor and a myoma. A gynecologist doing a pelvic exam asks herself, "What is this I am feeling here? Is it a myoma, an ovary, a cyst, or a tumor?" With her hands, she can feel whether it is close to the uterus and whether, when she moves the uterus, the excrescence moves with it. If so, the growth is most likely a myoma. If not, it can be a pedunculated myoma—a myoma attached to the uterus by a stalk—or it can be an ovarian tumor.

The main concern, of course, is whether the growth is cancerous. A myoma rarely turns into a leiomyosarcoma—the sarcomatous degeneration of a myoma—but it does occur in one-half to one percent of cases. This is why, if a patient has a myoma of any considerable size, she is asked to return for examination every six months (every year for a small size). Myomas are as slow-growing as slugs, and they can be monitored by repeat examinations. Their size is measured in comparison with pregnancy. The gynecologist writes on the patient's chart: "A 10-week-size uterus consistent with a myoma" or "A 14-week-size uterus consistent with a myoma." Patients speak of myomas as being the size of a lemon, orange, or grapefruit, but gynecologists do not.

Sometimes the uterus is the size of a 24-week pregnancy, the lady is 48 years old, she has a negative pregnancy test, and ultrasound testing shows no fetus in there. Tell that to an audience of gynecologists and obstetricians and they say, "Wow!" Tell that to the patient and she asks what it means. To establish some landmarks: A 12-week-size pregnancy is at the tip of the pubic bone, which is just under the bikini line. If the uterus goes above the pubic bone, it is a 14-week size. Once it starts to creep above the pubic bone, the gynecologist becomes concerned because the uterus should not be that big—normally it is the size of a small pear and weighs about $2^1/_2$ ounces. The patient is not bleeding, she has not noticed any interference with her bowels or with urination, but the uterus is enlarging, the myoma is growing, and this may be the rare myoma that becomes malignant. Now the gynecologist will keep track of its growth not only by touch but by ultrasound, for a good ultrasonographer can measure a myoma. Say that it is $6 \times 6 \times 8$ centimeters on first testing, and six months later it is still $6 \times 6 \times 8$. It has not grown and that is reassuring. But if the dimensions have changed to $10 \times 12 \times 14$, that is when the doctor says, "We need to go into surgery."

As likely as not, the patient replies, "You doctors always want to take out uteruses. I want a second opinion." The doctor never replies, "I'm concerned about cancer"; that is not something one says to a patient. Recently I had a patient come to my office who said she had had a hysterectomy, and when I asked why, she said it was because she had a myoma that was growing. I knew immediately that it was because the doctor suspected cancer, but the patient did not know that.

If you have had a myoma since you were 22 years old, and when you were pregnant it got a little bigger, and now you are 34 and it is 8-weeks-size, but then six months later it is 14-weeks-size, that is when you need exploratory surgery. If it is a 14-week-size when you are examined by a gynecologist you have not seen before, that gynecologist will follow you for two years to see if the size changes before recommending surgery because even sarcomatous tumors are slow-growing and are usually encapsulated within the myoma. Better still, he or she will ask for your records from your previous gynecologist—an excellent reason for taking them with you when you move. If you have your records, then the gynecologist will know whether the myoma is something new or the same old myoma that has been there since you were 20. If it is the latter, the anxiety level goes down considerably.

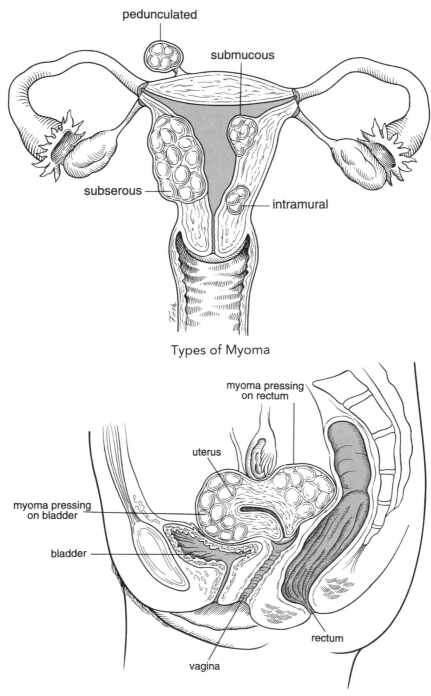

pepunculated

submucous

subserous

intramural

Types of Myoma

myoma pressing
on rectum

uterus

myoma pressing
on bladder

bladder

rectum

vagina

Interference of Myoma with Normal Function

If it is even larger than a 14-week-size—for instance, the size of a 16-week-pregnancy—and the previous records are not available, ultrasound testing is in order. Usually myomas are very firm and rubbery, and on ultrasound they can be seen projecting from the wall of the uterus on the inside or outside. All myomas start inside the thick wall of the uterus (intramural), with some growing out like Mickey Mouse ears (subserous) and some growing in (submucous), and it is reasonably easy to identify them. On the other hand, if a growth is large, it may be impossible to distinguish a myoma from ovarian cancer, in which case it is necessary to err on the side of caution and schedule exploratory surgery.

The patient's options are discussed with her before surgery, although if the growth proves to be malignant, she has none: A gynecological oncologist is called in and we do what we have to do to save her life. But if the growth should prove to be a myoma, we ask the patient whether she wants us to preserve her ability to have children or whether it is all right with her if we remove the uterus en bloc. If she opts for a myomectomy, we have to enucleate each myoma, shelling it out like a pea from a pod. Unfortunately, at the base of each myoma is the blood supply that has been feeding it, and the base bleeds copiously, requiring suture after suture after suture to stem the blood loss. If the myoma has grown deep into the uterus, the cavity of the uterus must be opened to get at it, so if the woman later has a child, it will have to be delivered by cesarean section because of the danger of uterine rupture.

Because there is so much blood loss associated with a myomectomy, sometimes a medication known as Lupron is given for a few months before surgery. Lupron brings on a mini-menopause that in some, but not all, instances shrinks the myoma. When the Lupron does work, the surgery goes better, but if the Lupron has not had the desired effect, the surgeon is clamping and cutting and tying and suturing while the blood continues to ooze. The bleeding is not the running stream of a hemorrhage but the oozing swamp of wetlands, and the uterus looks like a piece of Swiss cheese when the operation is over.

If the patient is 22 years old, all the difficulties of the surgery are worth it in order to preserve her reproductive capability. But if she is 42 and has two children and does not plan to have more, it makes no sense to do a myomectomy because it poses a far greater risk to her health than a hysterectomy. Myomectomies have the reputation of being a less invasive, less radical procedure, but that is not really the case. For one thing, there is no guarantee that the myomas will not grow back. For another, the bowel, which normally slides on the smooth surface of the uterus, may now stick to all the sutures that have had to be put in. The patient cannot pass gas, the bowel becomes obstructed, and there has to be repeat surgery to do a colostomy.

Resectoscopy. The younger woman should know—and ask her surgeon about—a new operative approach called resectoscopy. This involves going in through the cervix, viewing the inside of the uterus with a hysteroscope, and shaving off the growth hanging there with the resectoscope. At the same time the myoma is shaved, the area is cauterized, which prevents bleeding. Resectoscopy circumvents abdominal surgery for the young patient, but it requires a skilled person who has done many, many resectoscopies because it is all too easy to perforate the uterus or burn away vital areas.

Resectoscopy is only indicated if the myomas are inside the uterus. If they are on the outside, it may be possible to remove them laparoscopically, although not many doctors have the level of skill necessary to shave off the myoma, dissect it into very small pieces, and take the pieces out through the laparoscope. The majority of doctors prefer the more traditional approach because it allows them to look at all the other organs to see whether there is an ovarian problem or possibly adhesions; it also permits them to be certain that they have gotten the full extent of the myoma.

MYOMAS AND PREGNANCY

A woman who has a myoma can become pregnant, but because of the structural defect and the contour changes that come about with myomas, miscarriage is frequent. When a woman is an habitual aborter—defined as having had three or more spontaneous miscarriages—often the reason is that there is a big myoma in the uterus or the shape of the uterus has become distorted by myomas in the wall. If the myomas are subserous, that is, on the outside of the uterus, that is not an immediate problem because they are not where the baby is going to be growing. They are very likely, however, to cause preterm labor because now, with the placenta pumping out all that estrogen, which is a feast for the myomas, they grow larger and larger, and the uterus can only distend to a certain point. This is the case whether the uterus is being stretched by twins, triplets, or myomas. The uterus reaches its coefficient of expansion, and even if the pregnancy is only at 22 weeks, it sets about emptying itself with contractions.

There is no possibility of surgery for a myoma in a pregnant woman. If the blood loss is great in a nonpregnant woman, it is unthinkable in a pregnant woman because the tissues are soft and succulent and it is fiendishly difficult to do any kind of suturing. Surgeons tremble when required to operate on a pregnant woman even to remove an appendix or gallbladder. If it is a life-and-death matter, they have to, of course, but to do an "elective" myomectomy to reduce the size of a myoma is out of the question. Instead, the patient is put on bed rest, a high fluid intake, and tocolytic agents—such as ritodrine, terbutaline, and magnesium sulfate—to try to keep the irritability of the uterus down and get the pregnancy to at least 26 weeks and a viable baby.

Whether the patient is then delivered vaginally depends on where the myoma is. If it is on the outside of the uterus, you hope the vaginal birth will work because you do not want to have to go in through the abdomen for a cesarean and have myomas barring the way to the uterus. But you may have to do a cesarean because the baby is showing signs of fetal distress. You open the abdomen and there are these honkers with veins and arteries coursing all over them, a veritable road map of vascularity. You look at your assistant, take a deep breath, mutter, "I gotta go through. Get the clamps ready and hand them to me fast," and you cut.

In case you are now beginning to feel sorry for obstetricians like me who are faced with such situations, let me say that in medical school the brightest kids wanted to be internists and become elegant diagnosticians, but then we graduated and went out into practice and when we met again, the internists were saying, "The rest of my life I'll be seeing diabetics and doing vaccinations," while we obstetricians were saying, "Wow, every delivery is different, and what great babies!" Even though the hours are terrible, obstetrics is exciting, really a rush, and when the internists realize that, any number go back and do residencies in OB/GYN.

HYSTERECTOMY FOR MYOMAS

The indications for a hysterectomy for a myoma are a matter of common sense. If the patient is in her 40's or 50's, and if she is bleeding and bleeding, soaking a pad an hour during her periods and has clots, and if a trial of medication with progesterone or Provera has done nothing to remedy the situation, then she needs a hysterectomy. Another indication is the enlarging of the uterus beyond the size of a 12-week pregnancy. With a 14-week size the concern grows that a malignancy may be present, and if that 14-week size becomes a 16-week size, it is really incumbent on the gynecologist to do exploratory surgery to determine whether the size is due to a myoma, myosarcoma, or ovarian cancer.

As discussed, for a young woman who does not want to abandon the hope of having children, a myomectomy, even with all its problems, is the way to go. But if the patient has completed her family, a hysterectomy is the rational choice. Unfortunately, because of cultural influences, the uterus has become bound up with questions of identity and many a woman fears that she will be less female if this organ is removed. At this juncture I begin saying things like: "Okay, but you have a 16-week-size uterus and when I first saw you, it was 10-week-size, and that makes me nervous." I then break my own rule and mention the unmentionable. "I'm concerned that this is not just a benign situation, that we may be heading into a malignancy."

That gets the patient's attention, but still she protests: "My sister had a myoma this big and nobody mentioned malignancy."

"I'm not your sister's doctor and I was not there to know what was said. All I know is that a myoma is usually slow-growing but within a period of two years, this one has gone from a 10- to a 16-week size. Whether or not we are going to do a hysterectomy is up to you, but you're 45, you've had your three children, why do you need this dysfunctional organ?"

She may still not agree, and because of the heavy bleeding, her hematocrit keeps dropping, she is taking iron pills and they are making her constipated, and she is not enjoying intercourse because the myoma is butting against an ovary, which is truly painful. Finally, the situation so deteriorates that she has to capitulate and we do the surgery. What I hear then is: "Why didn't I do this three years ago? I feel so much better. I'm not constipated. I'm urinating better, and I don't have all that bleeding and clots. I wish I hadn't waited so long."

Sometimes I believe we gynecologists are not forceful enough advocates for what we know to be the right treatment. We allow a woman whose health is being undermined by excessive bleeding, and perhaps jeopardized by an undiagnosed malignancy, to refuse an operation because we are not strong enough to say flatly, "This is what needs to be done." Particularly are my male colleagues reluctant to pressure a female patient to have a hysterectomy because they do not want to be seen as sexist, but patients, too, need to take responsibility for their health and recognize when the signs indicate that a sensible rather than an emotional reaction is in order.

POINTS TO REMEMBER

- *Fibroid* is a misnomer. The correct term is *myoma*.
- One in every four women—one in every two black women—have myomas.
- Ask your doctor the size of the myoma and its location.
- A size greater than that of a 12- to 14-week pregnancy means trouble.
- Excessive growth of a myoma during the period of a year is a bad sign.
- One percent of myomas are cancerous.

17

ENDOMETRIOSIS

❧

DIAGNOSIS • MEDICAL TREATMENT • SURGICAL
TREATMENT •

Endometriosis is a disorder affecting young women in which endometrial tissue, normally serving only as the lining of the uterus, is scattered elsewhere. In some 10 percent of women between the ages of 25 and 50, islands of endometrial tissue are present in various other locations outside the uterus. The most common location is the pelvis, but endometriotic implants may also be seen on the ovaries and in the rectum, vagina, appendix, and bladder, even in episiotomy scars, the umbilicus, and such distant sites as the lungs. The condition may manifest itself as severe menstrual cramps (dysmenorrhea), chronic pelvic pain during a period, or painful intercourse (dyspareunia); or the only sign may be infertility; endometriosis is, in fact, the most common cause of infertility in women over 25. Since in endometriosis the islands of tissue are outside the uterus, the condition cannot be diagnosed by means of a traditional D and C, and visual inspection of the pelvic organs by means of laparoscopy must be done.

In endometriosis the ectopic or "renegade" uterine tissue has the same receptors for hormones as the uterine lining itself and responds in the same way. Cyclic changes in these cells during the menstrual cycle result in localized bleeding and inflammation in the ectopic endometrial tissue on the different organs, and these changes lead to the formation of adhesions. These adhesions are composed of dense scar tissue between one organ and another, making laparoscopy akin to being in a jungle with vines as thick as ropes entwined with one another. In order for the laparoscopy to proceed, these adhesions have to be cut, and done so without injury

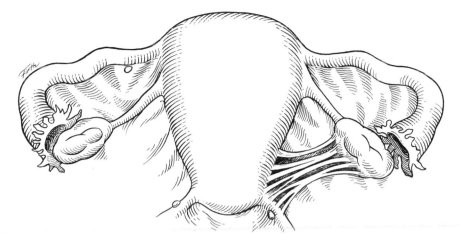

Mild Endometriosis: Shallow Implants, Filmy Adhesions

to vital organs, such as the bladder or bowel, which can readily be perforated or damaged during the procedure. Many an experienced cancer surgeon has been known to say that he or she would rather perform extensive, radical cancer surgery than have to deal with endometriosis.

No one knows exactly how endometriosis begins, but one prominent theory has it that in some women the menstrual blood not only exits via the cervix but also flows back up through the fallopian tubes and out into the abdomen. With each menstrual cycle, this spillage occurs again, unless pregnancy intervenes or the use of oral contraception results in a diminished flow. As can be surmised, delayed childbearing and not using birth control pills place a woman at higher risk for the development of endometriosis.

DIAGNOSIS

When I was a resident in training, the majority of young gynecologic patients who came to the emergency room with severe pelvic pain had one of two diagnoses: pelvic inflammatory disease or endometriosis. The working diagnosis was pelvic inflammatory disease if the woman was black and endometriosis if she was Caucasian, but since that time, studies have shown that endometriosis occurs

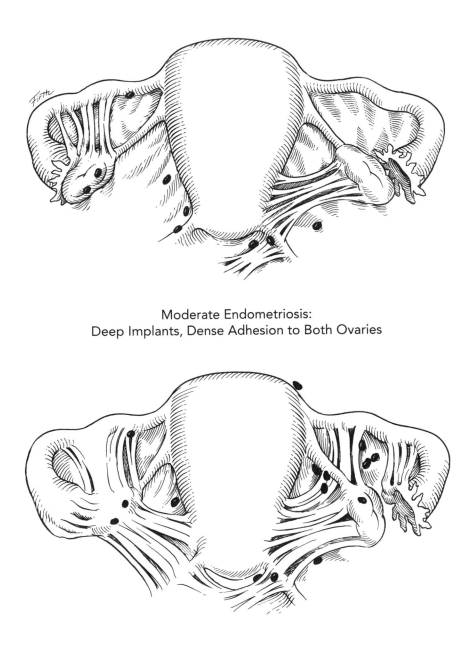

Moderate Endometriosis:
Deep Implants, Dense Adhesion to Both Ovaries

Severe Endometriosis:
Deep Implants, Dense Adhesions Throughout Pelvis

with equal frequency in all races. Therefore, if the patient is a woman of color but does not have the risk factors for pelvic inflammatory disease—sexually transmitted disease, multiple partners, frequent sexual activity, or history of IUD use—endometriosis should be considered in the diagnosis and the patient should be offered, rather than a short course of antibiotics, a diagnostic laparoscopy.

The first step in diagnosis is the taking of a detailed history coupled with a thorough, comprehensive pelvic examination, including a rectovaginal examination (see chapter 2). Patients can be immensely helpful to their physicians by completing a "pain map" identifying the locations where pain exists. The map divides the body into grids, and the patient writes an estimate of the pain level, from 1 to 10, in the appropriate box.

Once endometriosis has been diagnosed, treatment can be medical or surgical or a combination of both.

MEDICAL TREATMENT

Oral contraceptive medication (a combination of estrogen and progesterone), taken continuously, creates a pseudopregnant state by stopping the menses, and if the menses are stopped, reflux of the menstrual flow back through the fallopian tubes does not occur. On the other hand, it may be sufficient for the Pill to be taken as it would be for contraception alone because this reduces the volume of menstrual blood and thus the likelihood of reflux. Sometimes progesterone alone is given; this reduces the pain associated with endometriosis but may lead to frequent "breakthrough bleeding," that is, bleeding throughout the cycle.

For many years the mainstay of endometriosis treatment was Danazol, a synthetic hormone with male (androgenic) properties. Danazol blocks the normal midcycle surge of FSH and LH (see chapter 1) and stunts the growth of the uterine lining directly. The side-effects are weight gain, swelling, decreased breast size, acne, vaginal dryness, change in sleep patterns, and deepening of the voice. A baritone voice is not a bad side-effect if you want to sound sexy, but take note that the voice change may be permanent.

Lupron (leuprolide acetate) is another medication used in endometriosis. This is a synthetic form of the gonadotropin-releasing

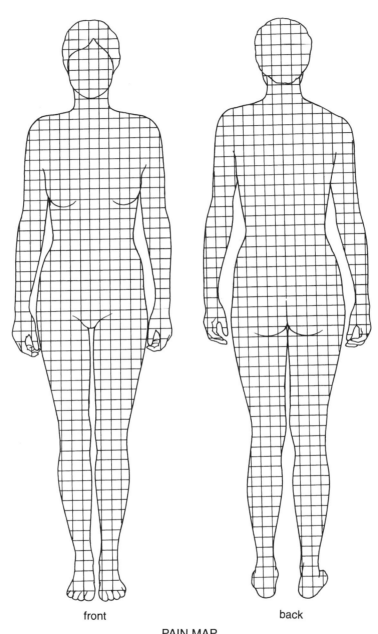

front   back

PAIN MAP

Grade the degree of pain from least (1) to most (10) intense, then
place number in appropriate corresponding grid square on map.

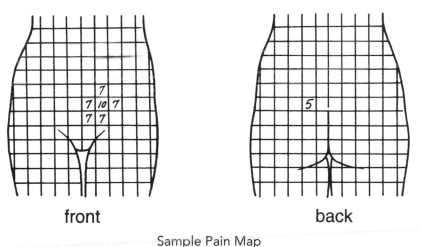

front   back

Sample Pain Map

hormone found in the hypothalamus, and it interferes with the pro-duction of FSH and LH by the pituitary gland. Without FSH and LH the ovaries stop producing estrogen and progesterone and men-struation ceases. The uterine lining shrinks and a pseudomenopausal state is created. The pain associated with endometriosis is relieved in most patients by the second or third month, which may or may not compensate for the possible side-effects of hot flashes, depression, headaches, mood swings, and loss of bone mineral density.

SURGICAL TREATMENT

At the time of a diagnostic laparoscopy, the endometrial implants may be surgically removed, cauterized, or vaporized with a laser beam. The cutting of adhesions can also be performed through the laparoscope, but if the implants are very large, if they cannot be reached by the laparoscope, or if organs such as the bladder and intestines are involved, abdominal surgery (laparotomy) is necessary. Both these procedures are considered to be conservative and are designed to protect the patient's childbearing capability and to cor-rect infertility if it is present.

The definitive treatment for severe, intractable endometriosis that does not respond to conservative management is a hysterectomy with removal of both ovaries. However drastic this may sound, it is necessary for women who have become pelvic cripples. They have had to endure unrelenting pain for so many years that the hysterectomy comes as a welcome relief. Hormonal replacement with estrogen is given, but not until three to six months after the surgery for fear it may trigger a reappearance of the disease. Progesterone is used with some patients to suppress any residual disease.

Even after a hysterectomy with removal of both ovaries, the endometriosis can recur, but it does so only in a very small number of patients. After medical therapy the recurrence rate runs as high as 50 percent; after laparoscopy it can be as high as 40 percent. Thus, compared to the other forms of therapy, hysterectomy, the most radical treatment, is also the most curative.

POINTS TO REMEMBER

- Endometriosis is the presence of endometrial tissue, which normally lines the uterus, in locations outside the uterus. It occurs in approximately 10 percent of women.
- Since the tissue responds to hormonal influence just as the uterine lining does, it causes bleeding, which in turn gives rise to pain, scarring, and adhesions.
- Endometriosis is the most common cause of infertility in women over 25.
- Medical treatment, which is hormonal in nature, can be helpful, but recurrences are common.
- Conservative surgical treatment is by means of laparoscopy or laparotomy.
- A hysterectomy is the most radical surgical treatment but also the most curative.

18

VAGINAL INFECTIONS AND SEXUALLY TRANSMITTED DISEASES

❧

VAGINAL INFECTIONS • BACTERIAL VAGINOSIS • YEAST INFECTIONS • URINARY TRACT INFECTIONS • GONOR-RHEA • SYPHILIS • HERPES • CHLAMYDIA • GROUP B *BETA*-STREPTOCOCCUS • TRICHOMONAS • HIV •

VAGINAL INFECTIONS

Do not treat an itch or discharge by yourself. Consult a gynecologist. Do not douche beforehand and go armed with the knowledge that the only way the gynecologist is going to find out what is causing the vaginal infection is by means of a culture to identify the organism or a wet smear with potassium hydroxide to identify the fungus. If the organism is not identified, then treatment is a shoot-from-the-hip approach of, "Try this and if it doesn't work, we'll try that." Whatever is prescribed—whether it is vaginal creams, sulfa drugs, or local antibiotics—changes the milieu of the vagina so that the organism later identified after the patient has come back and back may not be the same organism that originally caused the problem.

The culture goes to a commercial laboratory for a panel of tests that should include chlamydia, mycoplasma, and ureaplasma, and tests for fungus and gonorrhea. I have heard doctors say, "Oh, we don't do GC cultures in my office. My patients don't have gonorrhea." My answer is, "How do you know they don't if you don't do a culture?" If the patient is having intercourse and cannot be absolutely certain that the relationship is mutually monogamous, gonorrhea is one of the possibilities that has to be considered. If the woman is certain that she and her partner are mutually monogamous but then she develops a discharge and the culture identifies chlamydia or gonorrhea . . . well, that is when the gynecologist does a few somersaults. The patient is crying and saying, "How can that be?" and I as the gynecologist am not about to break up a family, so I tell her, "Oh, it's from a public bathroom. It's from towels. It's from swimming. It's from . . ." whatever I can make up. I know what it is from; it is from screwing around, but I can't say that.

The risk of getting a venereal infection depends on the lifestyle of the individual and her partner. If the woman is not monogamous or if she cannot be sure that her partner is monogamous, she should have a complete panel of tests once a year. There are stages to all the venereal diseases, and early diagnosis and treatment are important. People say, "Oh, I'll get to it. I'll get to it," then the initial symptoms clear and they forget about it, but that is unwise, for the consequences can be serious.

Bacterial Vaginosis. Bacterial vaginosis (BV) is currently the most common form of vaginal infection in women of childbearing age and has recently been identified as a cause of preterm births.

This vaginal infection has had six different names during the past one hundred years, which is a dead giveaway that its cause and treatment have been little understood. In this condition, the normally abundant lactobacilli, the good bacteria, are replaced by an overgrowth of the anaerobic bacteria that are usually present in only small numbers in the vagina. The prime symptom is an unpleasant fishy odor, especially after intercourse; the odor is due to the release of trimethylamine, a byproduct of the breakdown of the anaerobic bacteria. The recommended treatment is with Flagyl, either orally or in a vaginal gel. Conservative physicians treat both partners even though the CDC does not recommend this procedure as routine. Before prescribing Flagyl, the doctor will inquire about alcohol use, seizure history, and gastrointestinal problems because these can cause difficulties in connection with Flagyl.

Yeast Infections. Yeast, fungus, and *Candida* are interchangeable terms. Unlike BV, a yeast infection is not bacterial and cannot be treated with antibiotics; instead, it is a type of fungus, like athlete's foot, and must be treated with antifungal medication. The second most common vaginal infection, three out of four women will suffer from it at one time or another; the number of such infections doubled between 1980 and 1990. The symptoms are a cottage cheese–like vaginal discharge and severe itching, which can be the source of acute discomfort and embarrassment in an office or social setting. There are four main causes of a yeast infection: douching, the use of antibiotics, diabetes, and pregnancy. If the infection is recurrent and resistant to the usual treatment, HIV infection must also be considered.

The yeast infections are caused by one of many types of fungus called *Candida*. *Candida albicans*, the most common offender, is exquisitely sensitive to the class of drugs known as imidazoles (Monistat, Femstat, Mycelex). These medications became very popular in the 1970s and 1980s because of their ease of use and effectiveness against *C. albicans*. Unfortunately, they are not effective against *C. glabrata*, *C. tropicalis*, *C. krusei*, or *C. parapsilosis*.

In the 1950s, a dark purple liquid known as gentian violet was in common use for yeast infections. It was highly effective, but it permanently stained everything it came into contact with—examination tables, white coats, underwear, patient gowns, fingers, instruments—causing a general mess. However, with the return of some resistant fungal infections, use of it is resuming, this time in capsule form. Also useful for vaginal insertion in capsule form is boric acid. It should be noted, though, that oral sex and boric acid do not mix. If boric acid is accidentally swallowed, it can prove fatal.

In my travels, I have heard of many home remedies for vaginal yeast infections, from boiling one's underwear in order to kill off the spores, to inserting garlic in the vagina, to the most popular one of putting yogurt in the vagina to bring up the level of good bacteria. Yogurt does have lactobacilli present, although only in small amounts, but it is very high in natural sugar, and since yeast thrive on sugar, treating a yeast infection with yogurt is akin to spreading weedkiller in your garden but then adding fertilizer; you are defeating your purpose.

The newest treatment for yeast infections is the family of drugs known as triazoles (terconazole and fluconazole). These medications demonstrate some activity against the non-albicans species of *C. krusei*, and they appear to be more potent than the imidazoles against *C. albincans*. Terconazole is formulated for local vaginal application, while fluconazole is taken orally. Since the side-effects of the latter include possible liver damage, this oral antifungal medication should be taken only as a last resort.

Urinary Tract Infections. Urinary tract infections very often go hand in hand with vaginitis. The vagina and rectum are filled with naturally occurring and necessary bacteria, but the urethra, which enters the bladder, is sterile; urine is sterile. If any contamination travels from the vagina to the urethra, the result is a urinary tract infection, or cystitis, which causes painful urination or inability to urinate at all. "Honeymoon cystitis" is particularly common because initial intercourse causes trauma, so bacteria can readily be dispersed from the vagina to the urethra. Cystitis is treated with a broad-spectrum antibiotic—that is, one that is effective against a broad spectrum of organisms. The only problem with treatment is that the antibiotic sometimes eradicates not only the bacteria in the urethra and bladder but elsewhere in the body, and when the bacteria are gone from the vagina, fungus may move in. The street wisdom is that you should consume yogurt made with live cultures to head off fungal, or yeast, infection, but there is no evidence to suggest that doing this makes the slightest bit of difference.

The same is true of cranberry juice, which is reputed to be useful in urinary tract infection. Cranberry juice is acidic and it may help lower the pH slightly, but no studies have been done that prove it makes a difference. What does make a difference is plain water, eight glasses a day. If a woman drinks that much water, her urine is diluted instead of concentrated, and it is concentrated urine that predisposes to cystitis. Admittedly, it is not easy to drink eight glasses of water a day, but if you drink water instead of soda or tea or coffee or orange juice, which do not substitute for water in your body, it can be done. I recommend this plan: Chill two quarts of water in the refrigerator; take one to work with you and drink it during the day; when you get home at night, drink the other quart, then fill both bottles back up to chill for the next day. Every patient of mine who follows this regime becomes considerably less vulnerable to urinary tract infection.

GONORRHEA

Gonorrhea, one of the oldest sexually transmitted diseases known to man, is caused by the bacteria *Neisseria gonorrhoeae*. It presents in women as a persistent discharge that may be green and may be malodorous, but in any case is different from any discharge the woman is accustomed to. This is another of those instances in which you have to be attuned to your body to recognize that something out of the ordinary is going on so that you can seek prompt diagnosis and treatment.

Diagnosis is made by culturing the organism. If the culture is positive for gonorrhea, both partners must be treated to obviate reinfection. Treatment is with penicillin and is important because the infection can cause havoc with the ovaries and tubes, leading to sterility and perhaps necessitating a hysterectomy because of adhesions inside the pelvic cavity.

In women the site where material for the culture is obtained is the cervix. However, the highest rate of positive cultures comes from the pharynx and the anus, and if the cervical culture is negative for gonorrhea but the discharge persists, then a culture from one of these sites may give a positive reading. In men with "the drip" or "the clap," the culture material is taken from the penile urethra.

The gynecologist's problem lies in knowing that both sexual partners must be treated but having only one in the office. My solution is to write a prescription for penicillin sufficient to treat both and indicate to the pharmacist, "This is for Mary Jones and for her partner Henry Brown, *unless* Henry Brown is allergic to penicillin." Without the disclaimer, if Henry Brown has an anaphylactic reaction and I am the physician who signed the prescription, I am in a lot of trouble. This kind of dual prescription seems to me the most expeditious way of seeing to it that partners get treated, but it is perfectly possible, of course, that the gentleman may deny he needs treatment, saying, "I've never been cultured. It's not me." It is up to the woman then to answer firmly, "I have it, I've had sex with you, you have it. Period." She really has to insist; otherwise, she will be reinfected and the whole cycle will start over again.

On the whole, this all sounds easy: you get gonorrhea, you take penicillin, you are cured, and that was indeed the way it was until 1976 when penicillin-resistant *Neisseria* made their appearance, primarily around military bases. Prostitutes in the Philippines, say, routinely got their shots of penicillin, and the original gonorrhea that was very sensitive to penicillin began to adapt to it and became sensitive no longer. Now if we find that the gonorrhea is penicillin-resistant, we have to go to other methods of treatment. Spectinomycin, which belongs to the family of tetracyclines, is used, or ceftriaxone, or another type of antibiotic called cephalosporin. Indeed, penicillin-resistant gonorrhea is now so widespread that often penicillin is not even tried and these other drugs are used first.

A total of about one million cases of gonorrhea are reported annually, with the highest incidence among women occurring in the 20 to 24 age group. Insistence on the use of condoms lowers the risk of infection, just as with HIV, but nothing is one hundred percent effective. Condoms can come off in the midst of intercourse, or the condom might not come totally over the shaft of the penis and some spillage occurs that allows the bacteria to get through.

SYPHILIS

It used to be that you could not get a marriage license in most states without first being tested for syphilis. Now that that is no longer a requirement, the incidence of syphilis is increasing by leaps and bounds because it is easy to ignore the initial symptom of a small genital lesion that appears after an incubation period of 10 to 90 days. The lesion, which is called a chancre, can be on the cervix or vulva and persist for two to six weeks. Then it heals and disappears, and the only clue to the syphilitic infection is swollen lymph nodes, particularly in the groin.

If not detected and treated, the infection continues to the stage of secondary syphilis, which usually appears in the form of a skin rash, often on the palms of the hands. This secondary stage is highly infectious. (Since only one major infection causes sores on the palms and that is secondary syphilis, I would suggest that you not shake hands with someone with palmar lesions.) Another manifestation of this stage may be condyloma lata, little wartlike projections in the perineal area. These lesions may last a few months, then disappear, and the syphilis progresses to the third stage, where it can affect the central nervous system, all without the person realizing that he or she is infected because they have never had a culture.

The first indication of syphilis may be an unexplained stillbirth. In a search for the cause, blood is drawn and is tested for the offending organism, the spirochete *Treponema pallidum*. If present, it can explain the occurrence of preterm labor and neonatal death.

The treatment for syphilis is, again, penicillin, 2.4 million units given in a single intramuscular injection, or if the patient is allergic to penicillin, erythromycin or tetracycline. If the syphilis is of more than one year's duration, 2.4 million units are given weekly for three weeks. If the infection has reached the nervous system, penicillin is given intravenously for two weeks, then intramuscularly once a week for three weeks.

HERPES

Another sexually transmitted disease is herpes. Because herpes is a virus that sets up housekeeping along the neural pathways in the body, it cannot be cured, only its symptoms alleviated. The virus causes fluid-filled lesions on the vulva that are single or multiple and mild to severe. Like a fever blister on the lip, the lesions are tiny grapelike clusters, and the pattern of healing is the same as on the lip: You have the blister, it ruptures and is painful, then it starts to heal with a scab, which later comes off.

Sometimes the lesions are so painful that the woman gets to the point where she is afraid to urinate. The urinary flow contacting the lesions hurts so fiercely that she allows her bladder to become overdistended and she must be catheterized, even hospitalized and an indwelling catheter put in place until there has been some healing.

A palliative treatment for herpes is to sit in the bathtub and pour Betadine over the lesions—the solution, not the soap—straight out of the bottle. Then you turn the bathwater on and just sit there with your bottom in six inches of water. If at all possible, you do this three times a day; if not, before you go to work and before you go to bed. That basically makes the lesions more bearable; you can live with them for the seven to ten days it takes for them to run their course. A strong word of caution: The tub must be scrubbed out with Clorox afterward to eradicate the virus-shedding particles that can transmit herpes to a roommate or partner.

The virus is highly contagious, and because it cannot be eradicated and flares up again and again from a dormant state, men and women should tell their sexual partners that they are prone to having the virus and condoms must be used. Even someone not at the active stage may very well be shedding virus. It is conceivable that herpes can be picked up from a toilet seat if the little bullous lesions harbored by the previous occupant have just ruptured, and it is even more possible to contract herpes in a communal hot tub. In fact, a lot of infections that we never thought could be transmitted other than sexually can be passed around in a hot tub. The little bacteria hit the hot water, say "Oooh, this is great!" and travel happily from Susan to Michael to Jane to Robert.

Because herpes and syphilis both cause lesions, in order to make the differential diagnosis, material from the lesion must be cultured. The doctor takes a Q-tip, usually soaked with saline, and rubs it in the lesion to pick up cells, which is painful but necessary. When I hear from a patient that she has herpes, I ask how it was diagnosed. If it was done by means of a blood test, that does not mean much; anybody who has ever had a fever blister may have a positive antibody test. The diagnosis has to be made from the lesion itself to be sure it is type II, not just type I herpes—type I appearing on mucous membranes above the navel, type II below the navel, in the genital area.

Nowadays a laboratory can identify the virus very quickly with DNA probes. These probes are made of deoxyribonucleic acid (DNA), which is found chiefly in the nuclei of cells and carries genetic information. The probe basically has fragments to match herpes, and if the patient does not have herpes, the probe does not hook on. It is the same process with gonorrhea; the probe identifies and attaches to *Neisseria gonorrhoeae* if it is present.

Acyclovir, by now a well-known treatment for herpes, is best for initial outbreaks; it has little efficacy against further eruptions. However, if a patient has persistent and recurrent herpes, she and her physician may decide that she should best continue on oral therapy to try to head off or attenuate further attacks.

In the practice of obstetrics, it used to be routine to deliver the babies of women with a history of herpes by cesarean section because in 40 percent of cases of neonatal herpes the baby died. But then we found that the morbidity of the operative procedure was greater than the number of babies who developed herpes, so we decided to make the criteria more specific. If, at the time of labor, lesions are visible or if the mother had her last attack within a week of delivery, then she should have a cesarean section; but if the last attack was three months earlier and no active lesions are visible, then we feel it is sufficient to notify the neonatalogist of the mother's history so that the baby is quickly given acyclovir after it is born.

CHLAMYDIA

Chlamydia, an infection currently of epidemic proportions, is not a bacteria, not a fungus, not a virus, but an organism that is somewhere in between, like something out of Star Trek. It is referred to as an energy parasite because the organism lacks the enzyme systems that would enable it to generate its own energy, making it dependent on the host cell for energy and nutrition.

This organism can cause pneumonia in children, sterility and infertility in males, and pelvic inflammatory disease in females that may so damage the fallopian tubes and ovaries that a woman becomes unable to conceive. It can cause mothers to go into preterm labor, and if a baby is born with chlamydia, it does not fare well because its lungs are infected. The baby may become very ill and die, or it may have to remain hospitalized for a long period of time while it is being treated for chlamydia pneumonia.

No specific symptom signals the presence of chlamydia; there is no lesion as in syphilis, no voluminous greenish discharge as in gonorrhea, no painful outbreak of sores as in herpes. The infection is sexually transmitted, and because people do not know they have it, they readily pass it along, leading to about four million new cases each year, with an estimated one billion dollars in associated direct and indirect costs.

The site most usually affected by chlamydia is not the vagina but the cervix, which means that the woman seldom knows she has it unless she becomes concerned about a discharge. What the gynecologist sees on examination is that the cervix is swollen and red and has a whitish discharge. Culturing of that discharge identifies the infection. (In men the infection causes a nonspecific urethritis.)

The risk of getting chlamydia depends on the individual's lifestyle. If the woman and her partner are not mutually monogamous, or if she is monogamous but is not certain about her partner, she should be tested once a year. If she is certain but then she develops a discharge and the culture identifies chlamydia . . . well, as I say, that's when the gynecologist does verbal handsprings.

Chlamydia has become so widespread that, like gonorrhea and syphilis, it has to be reported to the Board of Public Health. The patient must give the name of all contacts, and the Board of Public Health gets in touch with them about treatment. The treatment recommended by the CDC is seven days of erythromycin; penicillin does not work well against chlamydia except as a second-line drug. After seven days the patient is tested again, and if the culture is still positive, treatment has to be repeated. Infertility specialists, because they are acutely aware of the impact chlamydia can have on fertility, tend to treat it more aggressively, using a six-week course consisting of four weeks of Vibramycin, which is a type of tetracycline, followed by two weeks of erythromycin (enteric-coated to protect the stomach). During this course the woman should not become pregnant because the tetracycline may affect the growing embryo.

GROUP B *BETA*-STREPTOCOCCUS

Another sexually transmitted infection is Group B *beta*-streptococcus, with the bacteria being passed back and forth between partners. It is not in the same league as chlamydia or herpes because it causes no problems unless the woman is pregnant. But if the woman is pregnant, the infection can cause premature rupture of the bag of waters, leading to preterm labor, and if the baby is delivered in the midst of Group B *beta*-strep, illness or death in the baby.

Urban areas, inner city areas, have high attack rates of Group B *beta*-strep. When it is identified by a positive culture, the patient is treated with penicillin, and we ask her to have her partner take penicillin, too. Sometimes the patient recolonizes after treatment—that is, the bacteria reappear in the vagina—and a second course of penicillin may be necessary. If the culture is still positive, we tell her not to worry about it, that it will not be a problem until, or unless, she goes into labor. At that point in time, she will be given antibiotics prophylactically to lessen the risk that the baby may pick up the infection.

TRICHOMONAS

Trichomonas is a parasite that causes a watery discharge and intense itching. The parasite is flagellated, meaning that it has lashlike appendages that propel it along. When a bit of the discharge is placed on a slide and put under a microscope, the swimming parasites are readily visible. The infestation is not life-threatening—it is not as bad as gonorrhea or chlamydia or syphilis, any one of which can affect the internal organs—but it is dreadfully uncomfortable.

The organism can be eradicated with an antiparasitic medication. Both partners need to be treated; otherwise, the organism is simply passed back and forth. Since the medication, Flagyl, has the same chemical structure as Antabuse, anyone taking it dare not drink alcohol without risking getting violently ill.

HIV

Human immunodeficiency virus, which is sexually transmitted, affects the immune system, and when a person's immune system is compromised, he or she becomes susceptible to many diseases that ordinarily could be fought off, from simple diseases like yeast infections to opportunistic organisms like herpes. Toxoplasmosis, lung infections, and everything else that the immune soldiers in the body would customarily do battle with and usually win out against can wander in and set up housekeeping because there has been a massacre of the soldiers.

The person whose immune system has been defeated will die, which is what is happening in ever-increasing numbers to women and children. The CDC has stated that: ". . . HIV (human immunodeficiency virus infection) has become a leading cause of morbidity and mortality among women, the population accounting for the most rapid increase in cases of acquired immune deficiency syndrome (AIDS) in recent years. As the incidence of HIV has increased among women of childbearing age, increasing numbers of children have become infected through perinatal (mother-to-infant) transmission. Thus, HIV has also become a leading cause of death for young children . . ."

If HIV had been handled early on in the same way as any other communicable disease, it would not have reached its present epidemic proportions. But because of the stigma attached to it, we did not say, "Okay, you have HIV, who are your partners? Let's get them in for treatment, or at least tell them about it so that they don't spread it to other people." When resistant strains of tuberculosis caused a resurgence of that infection, health departments all over the country beefed up their outreach programs, sending workers into shelters with the authority to say, "This is your medication. If you don't take it, you are going to be incarcerated, quarantined in jail." Without a similarly dispassionate approach to HIV, the epidemic can only get worse, with all levels of society affected, heterosexual and homosexual, young and old.

In the absence of an effective treatment of the virus, abstinence or mutual monogamy is the safest course. After that comes the use of condoms. This is a male prerogative but women should insist on it. The female condom (see chapter 4) is clumsy to use and sometimes the penis goes to the side of it, making it ineffective for both disease protection and contraception.

POINTS TO REMEMBER

- Both partners should be treated if one is found to have a sexually transmitted disease; if not, the infection will be passed back and forth.
- Gonorrhea causes a green and malodorous discharge.
- It is easy, but very dangerous, to ignore the initial symptom of syphilis: a small genital lesion that appears after an incubation period of 10 to 90 days.
- A rash on the palms of the hands can be a sign of secondary syphilis.
- Herpes, a virus, cannot be cured. Bathing with Betadine may be a way to relieve the pain of the fluid-filled lesions on the vulva that rupture. Afterward, the tub must be scrubbed with Clorox.
- Chlamydia, which has become a widespread epidemic, has no specific symptoms. People seldom know they have it unless tested for it. It can cause premature labor in pregnant women and serious illness in the baby.
- Group B *beta*-streptococcus is troublesome only in pregnant women, where it can cause premature labor and illness or death in the baby.

- Trichomonas is a parasite that causes a watery discharge and intense itching.
- HIV has become a leading cause of illness and death in women and their children. Abstinence or mutual monogamy is the first line of defense, use of condoms the second.
- Sexually transmitted diseases can be picked up in hot tubs.
- Prompt treatment should be sought for any venereal disease.

HYSTERECTOMY HYSTERIA

❧

A hysterectomy is defined as surgical removal of the uterus; -*ectomy* meaning to cut and *hyster-* a combining form referring to the uterus. The uterus is comprised of two parts: the fundus, which is the body of the womb, and the cervix, which is the mouth of the womb. Subtotal hysterectomies, in which the fundus is removed but the cervix is left in place, used to be common, but they were found to increase the risk of cervical cancer, so now both fundus and cervix are removed in what is referred to as a total hysterectomy.

Many woman assume that a total hysterectomy means removal of the ovaries as well, but the uterus and ovaries are two different reproductive sites and a total hysterectomy may very well leave the ovaries in place. Removal of the ovaries is known as a bilateral salpingo-oophorectomy, but since this is not an easy term to toss around, patients usually settle for saying, "I had a total hysterectomy," and the gynecologist has to inquire, "Do you mean your ovaries were removed also?" This fact is important to know because if the ovaries were removed, it impacts estrogen replacement therapy, hot flushes, and the patient's risk of heart disease and osteoporosis.

Unless there is some strong indication for their removal, the ovaries are allowed to remain in place if the patient is less than 40 years of age so that estrogen release continues. But if the patient is 45 or 50, I strongly urge that the ovaries be included in a hysterectomy because ovarian cancer is an insidious disease with no early warning signs, and to leave the ovaries in place is asking for

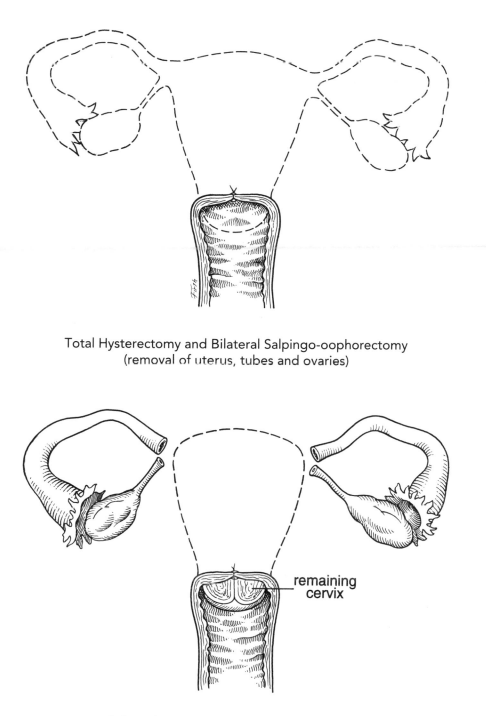

Total Hysterectomy and Bilateral Salpingo-oophorectomy
(removal of uterus, tubes and ovaries)

remaining
cervix

Subtotal Hysterectomy (cervix left behind)

trouble. Better that the patient go on estrogen replacement therapy a few years earlier than she would have with normal menopause. While there is more to ovaries than just the production of estrogen, there is also more to life than having ovarian cancer. If you are in your 40s and must have a hysterectomy for whatever reason, you should strongly consider having your ovaries removed at the same time. If it were me, I would insist on it, with absolutely no hesitation.

If the ovaries have been left in place after a hysterectomy, the patient may be surprised to discover that her breasts still get enlarged every month and she still has mood swings. This is because the ovaries and uterus are end-organs; they simply do what they are told by the pituitary and hypothalamus. It is not the uterus that causes menstrual bleeding and it is not the ovaries; it is the pituitary gland that gives out signals that say, "Oh, you're not pregnant this month? Well, the heck with it. Maybe next month"—and a period commences. Without a uterus present to do the bleeding, the period, of course, does not commence but still the messages come and still there are the premenstrual changes in response.

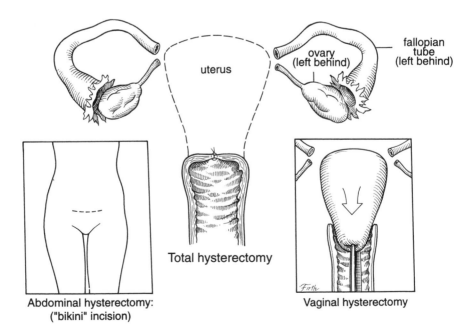

ovary (left behind) fallopian tube (left behind) uterus

Total hysterectomy

Abdominal hysterectomy: ("bikini" incision)

Vaginal hysterectomy

NECESSARY/UNNECESSARY HYSTERECTOMY

So much has been said and written about unnecessary hysterectomies that there is scarcely a woman who does not say "No, no" when a hysterectomy is recommended. An example: A woman comes into the office with a hematocrit in the low 30s (normal is between 35 and 42); she is becoming anemic because she is bleeding heavily every month. The next time I see her, her hematocrit has gone below 30, and the following time, despite iron replacement, it is at 25. I tell her we must start thinking about a hysterectomy, and she says, "I want to keep my uterus." I ask why, and the answer is because she wants to have children, though she admits she has not yet met the man she wants to have children with.

"Okay," I tell her, "you're 41. Say you take a year for meeting somebody and another year before you both decide it is going to last, so you are approaching 43 before you even think about having a baby. Meanwhile there are three years during which this abnormal uterus is going to pour out blood every month and you are going to feel ill and dragged out. Is a uterus that important to your life?"

"Oh, yes," she insists. And the answer will be the same if instead of being single and childless, the woman is married and has three or four children. Why? If a doctor said to either of these women, "You have a big growth on the side of your neck and we are going to have to remove it," she would instantly agree. If she had an abscessed lung or a diseased kidney, she would not hesitate to have the operation that would restore her health. But if the doctor says, "Look, you're hemorrhaging every month, the pressure on your bladder is making you miserable, and intercourse is painful. Let's take this thing out of there," she refuses because, as long as she has a uterus, "I'm still a woman. I can still have children."

Is the ability to have children all it means to be a woman? I believe not. I think the fact that we are nurturing, we are warm, we are insightful, that we bring a female perspective and intelligence to bear on situations is what makes us special and as valuable as our male counterparts, and these qualities are not dependent on having a uterus. I think as women we grossly underrate ourselves if we refuse a solution to our health problems on the spurious ground that a hysterectomy somehow reduces our worth as people.

Yes, there have been unnecessary hysterectomies. Perhaps at one time the operation was resorted to too frequently, but now women know the indications for a hysterectomy: monthly hemorrhaging, a myoma that is growing, difficulty in urination and/or defecation, anemia from the blood loss, irregular bleeding, painful intercourse, a suspicion of cancer. Women themselves can have a pretty good idea whether a hysterectomy is necessary or unnecessary, and if the signs are there, it is foolish to hesitate on emotional grounds.

Looked at in one way, the whole female reproductive tract is unnecessary. You need a heart, you need lungs, but you do not need a uterus. You certainly do not need it for sexual pleasure because enjoyment of intercourse hinges on the clitoris. In fact, a hysterectomy heightens the enjoyment of sex in premenopausal women because there is no longer apprehension about becoming pregnant.

The pathology report that comes back from the laboratory after a hysterectomy may indicate that the uterus itself was normal, allowing the inference to be drawn that this was an unnecessary hysterectomy. But the *function* of this uterus was terrible: The patient had so much trouble with her period, so much pain and heavy bleeding that she was miserable for years. Is that still an unnecessary hysterectomy? The patient herself does not believe so. She says, "This is the greatest thing that ever happened to me! How come nobody ever told me how wonderful it would be?"

Nobody ever told her for the same reason that women who have miscarriages do not tell people about it: for fear they will be thought of as less than a woman. If you dare to intimate that you are happy that your uterus is out, something is wrong with you; you are not a real woman. Society says you have to want to keep your uterus. I have had women tell me that they do not dare confide to their friends, or even their husband, how happy they are after their hysterectomy to have all the misery over and done with. But they tell me, and that is why I make the point to my fellow gynecologists in workshops and seminars that we should be more forthcoming in presenting our reasons for performing hysterectomies and that each surgery should be individualized on the basis of the patient's history and presenting symptoms.

In medicine there are certain protocols, that if this happens or these signs are present, this is the right course to follow. It is because we observe these principles and tenets that patients live. If we breach them, that is when trouble lies ahead, and unfortunately we breach them all the time in gynecology. We let a uterus bleed and bleed and bleed instead of dealing with it as straightforwardly as we would any other malfunctioning organ of the body because we are afraid to say firmly, "This is what needs to be done." That is politics, not medicine, and it is a disservice to the patient.

OPERATIVE APPROACHES

There are three different surgical approaches to performing a hysterectomy: transabdominal, transvaginal, and laparoscopically assisted vaginal hysterectomy. *Trans-* is a prefix that in this case means "through." Thus, the surgeon can go through the abdomen or through the vagina to remove the uterus. When gynecologists were not trained to operate in the abdomen, transvaginal hysterectomies were common and gynecologists were adept at them, but not many are anymore. Residents in gynecology and obstetrics still have to do a certain number of them in an accredited training program, but few feel confident enough about this approach after they get into private practice to develop a real skill at it, and skill is necessary because it is virtually blind surgery, with much of it done by feel. The surgeon has to go in and cut the support ligaments around the uterus without cutting the ureters. Gynecologists now in their 60s and 70s are very good at it, and complications are fewer and recovery time shorter than with an abdominal approach, but younger doctors tend to favor a laparoscopically assisted approach.

With a laparoscope, the ligaments holding the uterus in place can be visualized, and once they are cut, the uterus can be dragged out through the vagina. Because sophisticated laparoscopic instruments are used, the procedure is more expensive than the transvaginal procedure but offers the same benefits of fewer complications and shorter hospitalization and recovery times.

PROLAPSE OF THE UTERUS

It can happen that the ligaments holding the uterus in place can stretch or let go, so that the cervix moves down into the vagina. The smallest prolapse, first-degree uterine descensus, is usually noticeable only to the gynecologist, who introduces a speculum into the vagina and then discovers it will go in only so far because it is being met by the cervix at about the midportion of the vagina. With second-degree descensus, the cervix is as far down as the introitus, or entrance, of the vagina, and with third-degree descensus it is hanging out of the vagina, which is uncomfortable for the patient and interferes with her sitting and walking. Because the cervix is not meant to be exposed to the air, in third-degree descensus it becomes dessicated and dry, the tissues start to bleed, and infection becomes a strong possibility. Nevertheless, a surprising number of women do not seek treatment. "Oh," they say, "I just push it back in."

Childbearing is the leading cause of prolapse. It can also be due to obesity or to a chronic condition like asthma or bronchitis that gives rise to frequent coughing. Urinary incontinence is sometimes mistakenly attributed to a prolapse; a patient arrives at the office saying, "Well, I'm losing urine and my uterus is falling down." Examination reveals that the problem is a chronic urinary tract infection, and once it is cleared up, the patient is relieved of the symptoms of pressure and fullness.

With a relaxed pelvic outlet, the descending uterus may pull some of the other organs into the vaginal canal because it is so close to the bladder and the rectum. The result is a cystocele, a hernial protrusion of the bladder, or a rectocele, a hernial protrusion of the rectum. When the prolapse is first-degree, there is usually no particular problem, but in more advanced stages, there has to be a surgical repair or the patient must use a pessary.

Pessaries sound as old-fashioned as high-button shoes and buggy whips, but if it is possible to find a surgical supply store that still sells them, they are great for older women who resist the idea of surgery or are not good anesthesia risks. The pessary in most common use is called a doughnut pessary because that is what it looks like. The gynecologist deflates it, fits it in the vagina to hold the cervix in place, and then reinflates it. Because the pessary may erode the delicate mucosa of the vagina, it should be examined and changed every six months. Alas, not every patient is faithful about returning, and when such a patient finally does come back the vagina is eroded and infected and the smell would clear the worst head cold in a minute.

The pessary is not like a diaphragm that the patient can put in and take out herself. Also unlike the diaphragm, it impedes intercourse, which is why it is not used in young women. But older women who are widowed and not into dalliance often find it preferable to surgery.

If surgery is decided upon, a vaginal hysterectomy is a simple matter because the cervix and uterus are already in plain view and it is just a question of snipping the ligaments. When a patient tells me that she had a vaginal hysterectomy, I say, "Oh, did you have a uterine prolapse?" I know that the answer is almost certain to be yes because vaginal hysterectomies are rarely performed these days for any other reason. As noted, younger gynecologic surgeons prefer the laparoscopically assisted vaginal hysterectomy so that they can visualize the ligaments and be certain what they are cutting even though older surgeons chide them with: "By the time you get the laparoscope in so you can view the area, I can have the whole uterus out, with less bleeding and no problems."

KEGEL EXERCISES

Doing Kegel exercises after childbirth is thought to prevent a prolapsed uterus. Developed by a Dr. Kegel, the exercise is designed to strengthen the ligaments and muscles that have been stretched during childbirth. A simple exercise that can be done while waiting for a red light to change or watching television, it involves tightening up the muscles in the vagina and the muscles used to hold back urine, keeping them tensed for a few seconds, and then letting go, and repeating this over and over. Sometimes a patient says, "I do the Kegel exercise but I'm still losing urine and I still have this cystocele." I inquire how often she does the exercise and that reveals the problem; she is doing it two or three times a day when to be effective it must be done one or two hundred times a day in divided segments of twenty at a time. But given that there is a new baby to look after and half the time the woman is too busy even to brush her teeth, we see a lot of relaxed vaginal outlets, particularly in women with several children. Johnny arrives at 7 pounds, Mary arrives at 8 pounds, and the uterus arrives at 1 pound.

POINTS TO REMEMBER

- The indications for a hysterectomy are: monthly hemorrhaging, a myoma that is growing, difficulty in urination or defecation, anemia from blood loss, irregular bleeding, painful intercourse, or a suspicion of cancer.
- A uterus found to be normal on pathological examination does not mean the hysterectomy was unnecessary if the organ was the source of debilitating symptoms.
- A total hysterectomy refers to removal of the uterus and cervix. Unless there is a reason to the contrary, the ovaries are left in place in women under 40, removed in women over 45. Between 40 and 45, it is a judgment call.
- Prolapse of the uterus is treated surgically or with a pessary.
- Kegel exercises done after childbirth can be helpful in preventing prolapse of the uterus.

20

CANCER AND HEART DISEASE

༄

DETECTION • PAP SMEAR • UTERINE CANCER • TAMOXI-
FEN AND ENDOMETRIAL CANCER • OVARIAN CANCER •
INCIDENCE AND MORTALITY RATES IN CANCER • HEART
DISEASE • CHOLESTEROL LEVELS •

Cancer and malignancy are the same thing, so let us not be afraid to use the word *cancer*. Tests that give early warning of breast, cervical, and uterine cancer are available, which is why it is important to have a mammogram, a Pap smear, and a pelvic examination once a year. Cancer in any one of these locations is slow-growing—unlike, say, pancreatic cancer—so it is unlikely to be much advanced when it is detected and the chances of cure are excellent. The initial stage is called carcinoma *in situ*, meaning "in its original site," and progression from *in situ* to invasive carcinoma takes place only over many years. In cervical cancer, for instance, the progression goes from normal cells to mild dysplasia (abnormality), then to severe dysplasia where the cells get more angry-looking, then to cancer, and after that the cancer takes a long time to break through the basement membrane and invade neighboring tissues. It is not a question of a normal examination one year and a finding of cancer the next—or at least only in rare instances.

DETECTION

Although the American Cancer Society says that every three years is often enough for a Pap smear, that is based on the assumption that every technician is perfect and that laboratories never make a mistake and call a slide normal when there are early signs of a little bit of cancer. Occasionally, a mistake *is* made, and if you return for another Pap smear a year later, that mistake is going to be picked up while the cancer is still at a preinvasive stage; but if you wait three years, the cancer has been left alone much longer than it should have been. If I did not see this often enough in my own practice, I am sure I could talk myself out of a yearly visit to my gynecologist because I hate the examination just as much as any other woman. I could say to myself, "I do not have any pain, no abnormal bleeding, so why do I need to go?" The answer is that I need to go because it is the things you don't know about that can kill you. Suppose I have a cancer that will take ten years to go from noninvasive to invasive. If I go for an examination every year, I have ten chances to catch it; if I go only every three years, I have only three chances. Therefore, as noted earlier, every woman from the age of 18 until God takes her out of here should see her gynecologist at least once a year.

If you are on birth control pills or are using a cervical cap, a visit to the gynecologist more often is indicated because either of these may cause changes in the cell structure of the cervix. Because an unintended pregnancy will be more of a problem than any cellular changes associated with the use of the Pill or cervical cap, there is no reason to forgo using either of them, but the possible dysplasia should be dealt with by colposcopy or laser treatment just to be on the safe side.

Pap Smear. In a normal Pap smear the cells under the microscope look rather like a fried egg, with the nucleus of the cell being the yolk and the cytoplasm being the surrounding white. The ratio of nucleus to cytoplasm is 1 to 16, meaning that the nucleus is small in comparison to the wide cytoplasm. With dysplastic changes, the nucleus gets larger and the ratio gets smaller and smaller. The cell becomes ugly-looking. Based on the ratio of nucleus to cytoplasm, the dysplasia is classified as mild, moderate, or severe, and finally as carcinoma *in situ*.

UTERINE CANCER

Uterine cancer occurs most frequently in nulliparous women—women who have not had children—heavyset women, women who have diabetes, and women who are taking unopposed estrogen, that is, estrogen not counterbalanced by progesterone. Concerning the

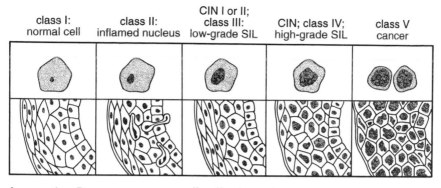

class I: normal cell	class II: inflamed nucleus	CIN I or II; class III: low-grade SIL	CIN; class IV; high-grade SIL	class V cancer

A negative Pap smear means all cells viewed are negative
A positive Pap smear means some cells are abnormal

Classification Systems:
SIL (squamous intraepithelial lesion), low-grade or high-grade, known as the Bethesda System (newest method); class I, II, III, IV, V (older method); or CIN (cervical intraepithelial lesion) I, II, III

latter, vaginal estrogen creams and the Estraderm patch are absorbed just as readily as oral estrogen, and progesterone is needed to protect the uterus.

Irregular bleeding is the usual presenting symptom in uterine cancer because cancer cells do not follow the rules of shedding once a month and not being heard from for another 28 days. Cancer cells say, "Ha! Every 28 days? You've got to be kidding. We'll shed whenever we want to and grow wherever we want to." The shedding may occur month after month or it may happen only once. If it is just once and the woman is not sufficiently attuned to the significance of irregular bleeding to consult her doctor, she may miss the single warning of the presence of uterine cancer.

Young women, in particular, and at the other end of the spectrum menopausal women, may have just the single episode of irregular bleeding. The definition of menopause is the absence of a period for six months, with 52 being the average age at which this occurs. Suppose you have had years of fun and frolicking, no periods, you can wear white pants any time you want, and then at 58 you start bleeding again. That is not the moment to go into denial, to say, "Oh, it's just my period. I got too excited or maybe I am coming down with a cold." Because the irregular bleeding may be a sign of endometrial cancer, it must be investigated. The cause may simply be a polyp, but then again it may not be or the polyp itself may be cancerous.

Tamoxifen and Endometrial Cancer. Tamoxifen, which is used in the treatment of breast cancer, is supposed to be an antiestrogen drug, but it has lately been recognized to have a modest estrogen effect too. Women had their breast cancer taken care of but then were found to be developing uterine cancer because, as noted by the American College of Obstetricians and Gynecologists, "this drug can induce or promote the development of a second primary neoplasm in the uterine endometrium of women with breast cancer."

The report goes on to state, "Annual gynecological examination and endometrial biopsies, plus transvaginal ultrasound, dilatation and curettage have been advocated." No woman wants to request any sort of invasive procedure, but for a patient taking tamoxifen, it is probably a wise course to request an endometrial biopsy once a year, as well as being alert herself for any sign of irregular bleeding.

OVARIAN CANCER

There are no early warning signs for ovarian cancer. Only a yearly gynecological examination detects its presence through changes in the size and shape of an ovary. It is estimated that 60 to 70 percent of all cases of ovarian cancer have reached an advanced stage of the disease, sometimes with liver metastases, by the time the patient presents to her physician.

In an attempt to devise an early warning system for ovarian cancer, investigators developed a monoclonal antibody to human epithelial ovarian carcinoma. Unfortunately, this screening test, known as CA-125, has not turned out to be as helpful as initially hoped.

Some interesting, albeit controversial, observations with regard to ovarian cancer have recently been published. One is that high dietary intake of animal fat is possibly associated with increased risk of developing the disease. Another is that investigators have noted that women who regularly dust their perineum with talcum powder and use talc on sanitary napkins have a threefold increased risk of developing ovarian cancer. And a third is that the greater prevalence of ovarian cancer in nuns, single women, and women who have never conceived suggests that continuous ovulation uninterrupted by pregnancy may also be a predisposing factor. It is of some interest that ovarian cancer is the commonest epithelial tumor in the best-known continuous ovulators: chickens. In addition, the incidence of ovarian cancer in hens is greatly increased when artificial means to enhance egg production are used.

In the United States it is estimated that the lifetime risk of developing ovarian cancer is one per 70 women (1.4 percent), and that one in every 100 women will die of the disease. On the positive side, use of oral contraceptive medications (birth control pills) confers protection against ovarian cancer, as, of course, does removal of both ovaries (bilateral oophorectomy). If a hysterectomy is being performed for any reason, many surgeons now advocate the prophylactic removal of normal ovaries in patients over 45, a position with which I agree, because the incidence of ovarian cancer increases significantly after the age of 40.

INCIDENCE AND MORTALITY RATES IN CANCER

Breast cancer is the most frequent cancer in women, with about 182,000 new cases a year, in comparison to ovarian cancer, at 21,000 new cases a year. But because there are no early warning signs or tests to detect ovarian cancer, the death rate is higher—about 62 percent in ovarian cancer, as opposed to 25 percent in breast cancer and 32 percent in cervical cancer. With the mortality rate in lung cancer at 80 percent, lung and ovarian cancers are thus the most lethal cancers in women, while breast and cervical cancers are the least.

(Lung cancer used to be thought of as a man's disease, but since the 1960s the incidence of lung cancer in women has risen 500 percent, while in men it has merely doubled. Smoking is the primary cause, of course.)

HEART DISEASE

The leading cause of death for women in the United States is not cancer but heart disease. Women account for 250,000 of the 550,000 deaths from cardiovascular disease each year. At younger ages, men are more likely to die of heart disease than women, but with increasing age, the death rate begins to even out. The risk factors for developing heart disease are smoking, high blood pressure, high cholesterol levels, diabetes, and obesity.

Estrogen levels are to some extent protective against heart disease in younger women, but with menopause, that protection fades and women are at equal risk. My own observation is that women are less likely to survive an initial heart attack than a man. Why? A woman is washing the dishes, say, and she has this pain in her chest. She says to herself, "The pain's not as bad as going into labor and having Joey, so it can't mean anything too serious." A man having the same degree of pain yells, "Oh, God, this is it! It's all over! Take me to the hospital!" But a pain has to be really debilitating in order to rivet a woman's attention, which means that by the time she gets to the emergency room at the hospital, her heart attack is at an advanced stage and she does not have as good a chance of recovering from it. If women were cognizant of the fact that chest and/or arm pain can mean a heart attack, rather than telling themselves that a heart attack is supposed to hurt a lot and the pain they feel is not as severe as when they had a baby, they would seek medical attention sooner and better their chances of surviving.

A second influence on women's survival rates can be a patronizing, paternalistic approach on the part of a male physician in the emergency room. If a woman over 50 says, "I'm having this pain," an unenlightened doctor may say, "It's probably menopausal. Here's some Premarin," and the woman dies in the parking lot on the way to her car.

What I am trying to illustrate is that we all, patients and physicians alike, need to have a heightened sense of awareness of the deaths associated with heart disease in women. If you go to an emergency room and a physician says, "Have a Valium, Mrs. Jones. You're just a little high-strung," you must as a patient say, "No, wait a minute, I want an EKG." You don't have to be belligerent or adversarial, but neither need you politely accept a Valium and go home. You must insist, "I have chest pain. I want an EKG." If the EKG is normal, the next thing to ask for is a determination of cardiac enzymes. When there is an obstruction of the heart muscle, cardiac enzymes in the blood give the first sign of it. If they, too, are normal, then accept the Valium and leave, but short of that, do not be intimidated if an emergency room nurse or doctor tells you, "We haven't got time for your pains. We have a gunshot wound over here and a broken ankle over there." Excuses are unacceptable, and valuable time may be lost in instituting treatment with the new drugs that dissolve clots in the coronary arteries if the diagnosis of heart attack is not made promptly.

Cholesterol Levels. As a causative factor in cardiovascular disease, the total cholesterol level is important, but not as important as the fractionated levels. You can have a cholesterol level of 250 and fear that you are going to die tomorrow, but if the HDL is high and the LDL is low, you are not in the slightest bit of danger. The higher the HDL level, the more protection you have against heart disease. It is LDL that deposits those plaques in your arteries that can kill you. I remember the difference by calling LDL the Lowdown Dirty cholesterol. You can have a total cholesterol level of 180, which sounds reassuringly low, but if the major part of it is LDL, there is trouble ahead.

POINTS TO REMEMBER

- Tests that give early warning of breast, cervical, and uterine cancer at a time when the prognosis is excellent are available and should be utilized yearly by every woman.
- For users of birth control pills or the cervical cap, more frequent gynecologic examination is recommended.
- Irregular bleeding can be a sign of uterine cancer.
- Tamoxifen, used in the treatment of breast cancer, may be a causative factor in uterine cancer.
- Since there is no really reliable test for ovarian cancer, a yearly gynecological examination is the best means of detection.
- Women using talc on the perineal area and/or on sanitary napkins are at increased risk of ovarian cancer.
- In women over 45, a hysterectomy should possibly include prophylatic removal of the ovaries even if they are normal.
- The leading cause of death in women in the United States is not cancer but heart disease.
- A woman experiencing chest pain should not ignore it, nor should she allow emergency room personnel to dismiss it. She

should insist on an EKG and, if that is normal, determination of the cardiac enzymes.

- LDL is the harmful type of cholesterol, while HDL protects against heart disease. Determination of each, rather than the overall cholesterol level, is what is important.

V

MENOPAUSE

21

MENOPAUSE

❧

PITUITARY HORMONES AND MENOPAUSE • HOT FLASHES AND FLUSHES • HORMONAL REPLACEMENT THERAPY • SIDE-EFFECTS AND CONTRAINDICATIONS • POST-HYSTERECTOMY • THE AGING PROCESS • HEART DISEASE AND STROKE • DEPRESSION • SKIN CHANGES • PAINFUL INTERCOURSE • OSTEOPOROSIS • POSTMENOPAUSAL BLEEDING • PSYCHOLOGICAL FACTORS • WEIGHT GAIN • PREMATURE MENOPAUSE • "OOPS" BABIES •

With the "graying" of the baby boomers in America, the number of menopausal women is increasing dramatically. It is estimated that currently, 4000 women each day enter menopause. By the end of the century, the life expectancy for women will be 82 years. Therefore, the average woman will pass 30 years (or about one-third of her life) after menopause.

In the United States, the average age of menopause is 52, with a range between 48 and 55. Menopause is defined as the complete cessation of menses for six months. After six months with no bleeding, if a woman is in the correct age group, she is considered menopausal. But this really means *no* bleeding. If spotting occurs at five months, she is still considered perimenopausal. Peri-menopause (also known as the climacteric) is the period of time immediately before and after menopause. It refers to the transition phase from the reproductive stage of life to a nonreproductive stage. The tent is being packed up, but the circus is not out of town until six spotless months have gone by. Just as menarche was a gradual process of breasts developing and hair growing under the arms, so, in reverse, is menopause a slow process of the time between periods spacing out, hot flushes coming on, and hairs sprouting under the chin.

These changes usually begin at about 48 years of age. A period that has been coming regularly skips a month, coming in March but not again until May, and after that perhaps not again until August, and the flow may be lighter. Each woman is different, but each knows the character of her own menses and will notice gradual changes in the timing and consistency over a period of four or so years. If she is keeping a menstrual calendar, as she should be, it will show at a glance the natural progression she is going through.

Some women sail through menopause. Some have a miserable time. Some are bedeviled by hot flashes and flushes, while some scarcely experience them. Some have cold flashes instead of hot flashes. Some women have chills following severe hot flashes. Some feel like ants are crawling all over their bodies, a sensation referred to as formication. Some suffer from depression, some from mood swings that may involve irrational anger or anxiety, some from listlessness and a loss of interest in activities they formerly enjoyed. But many women deal with menopause equably, knowing that it is in the natural order of things. Table 3 lists symptoms that can be associated with menopause, symptoms that may also occur in the perimenopausal period. Comparing symptoms with an informal support group of family members and/or friends who have been through the experience of menopause can be useful and reassuring. It is also helpful to have a physician who is a compassionate listener and will explain the pluses and minuses of treatment options.

TABLE 3

Symptoms Associated with Menopause

Physical	*Psychological*
Hot flashes and flushes	Insomnia, sleep disorders
Night sweats	Mood swings
Headaches (pressure, stress, migraine)	Depression
Cold feet and hands	Irritability
Numbness and tingling	Anxiety attacks
Formication	Forgetfulness (short-term
Joint pain	memory loss)

Physical	*Psychological*
Urinary incontinence	Inability to concentrate
Blind spots	Chronic fatigue
Heart palpitations	Decreased libido
Lightheadedness (dizziness)	
Feeling of suffocation	

Until recently, menopause has not been a socially acceptable topic of discussion, and women said to themselves that, along with childbirth, it was one more cross they had to bear. No more. Women born in the baby-boom years and now perimenopausal in the 1980s and 1990s are more assertive and are asking questions: "Why am I experiencing this? Is there something I can do? Why am I being given this medication? Is it a good idea to take it?" Doctors are having to enter into a dialogue about menopause, having to study up and attend symposia—to make up for the lack of attention paid to menopause in medical schools in the past—so that they can discuss the body's adjustment to the falling production of hormones and the fact that it is not an illness but a transition. It is becoming a learning experience for both physician and patient. The American Menopause Foundation, founded in 1993, is a nonprofit, independent health organization dedicated to providing support and assistance on all issues concerning menopause. It is located in the Empire State Building at 350 Fifth Avenue, Suite 2822, New York, N.Y. 10118 and can be called at (212) 714-2398.

PITUITARY HORMONES AND MENOPAUSE

In the years prior to menopause, estrogen and progesterone production decline despite continuing ovulation. With less estrogen, this stimulates the hypothalamus to increase the release of the gonadotropins, FSH (follicle-stimulating hormone) and LH (luteinizing hormone) by a negative feedback mechanism (see chapter 1). In the aging ovary, the remaining follicles become less responsive. Unlike the premenopausal ovary, which will produce estrogen and progesterone with a little coaxing from FSH and LH, the postmenopausal ovary does not respond as readily, resulting in low levels of estrogen with high levels of FSH and LH. High levels of FSH and LH, therefore, become markers in the blood that confirm whether or not a woman is menopausal and can be determined by a simple test.

When the estrogen production is low in the postmenopausal ovary, the major source of estrogen then becomes the adrenal gland, which converts adrenal androgens (male hormones) into a form of estrogen (estrone). Since this conversion is done in adipose (fat) tissue, overweight women have more circulating estrogen, which supports the observation that heavier women tend to have fewer of the menopausal symptoms that are related to low estrogen levels.

HOT FLASHES AND FLUSHES

The most common symptom of menopause is the dreaded hot flash or flush. The medical term for these two interchangeable words is vasoconstrictive imbalance. What happens until the body adjusts to the falling levels of estrogen is that the terminal ends of blood vessels undergo spasm. The hot flashes may occur months before the last menstrual period prior to the onset of menopause. About 85 percent of postmenopausal women have hot flashes, and about half of these women (45 percent) continue to have flashes for up to 10 years after menopause. The average flash, which lasts about 3 seconds, involves increased blood flow to the hands and skin—especially the skin of the face—and elevated temperature and pulse. This is followed by a sudden drop in body temperature and profuse perspiration over the affected area. This process may happen once a week, once a day, or many times a day. If the hot flash occurs during sleep, it is called night sweat. The intensity varies from woman to woman, but how a woman reacts to hot flashes and flushes also depends on her lifestyle.

As a physician, I have to take the woman's situation into account when deciding how I can best help her. If her work involves giving a lecture in front of two hundred people and her face turns scarlet, or if she is giving a presentation to a roomful of men and her silk blouse turns dark with perspiration, I think that it is important to her well-being that this lady receive estrogen replacement therapy to keep her on an even keel. After discussing the possible side-effects (see Table 4), she may willing accept my recommendation. On the other hand, if she is a grandmother, and has a hot flash while volunteering at the local library and another while shopping at the supermarket and is only momentarily miserable, she may not be a candidate for replacement therapy or may not want to take the medication after being told the side-effects. But if she tells me, "I get a little disoriented and don't know where I am for a while," then she and I may want to reconsider.

TABLE 4.

Side-Effects of Estrogen Replacement Therapy

Serious	*Less Severe*
Uterine cancer	Nausea
Blood clots in legs or lungs	Vomiting
Stroke	Water retention
High blood pressure	Breakthrough or irregular
Gallstones and gall bladder disease	bleeding
	Painful breasts (mastodynia)
	Weight gain

There are so many different types of women, and so many different types of situations women are in when they experience the flashes or flushes, and women differ so much in whether they are desperately embarrassed or can take them in stride, that treatment has to be individualized. My criteria are that if the menopausal symptoms are disruptive to a woman's quality of life or if she is at risk for osteoporosis, she needs to have hormonal replacement therapy. If her symptoms are mainly confined to hot flashes, Bellergal, a nonhormonal medication, may be the answer. Catapres (clonidine hydrochloride), a drug used to treat high blood pressure, has also been used successfully to reduce hot flushes significantly.

HORMONAL REPLACEMENT THERAPY

When a patient says, "I can't stand feeling like I'm hanging over hot coals by my thumbs. I can't live like this," many a harried doctor will write a prescription for Premarin and Provera and say, "Okay, Mrs. Jones, I'll see you in six months." If Mrs. Jones gets the prescriptions filled—which she may not do, because she has heard estrogen can cause cancer—she is then startled by the return of her period. "I didn't know this was part of the deal," she says. "I've had forty years of menstruating and I'm tired of bleeding every month." And her prescription, like many, many prescriptions for hormonal replacement therapy, is never refilled. It is estimated that 50 to 75 percent of women who start hormonal replacement therapy discontinue it within six months.

When a patient says, "I break out in terrific sweats in front of my students, and I wake up at night with my sheets soaking," I tell her, "You may be a candidate for hormone replacement therapy, but here's what it involves. It entails your taking medication for years, and each month you are going to have your period again. Along with the estrogen, you will be taking progesterone (Provera), which is what causes withdrawal bleeding and may also cause you to feel bloated, but without the progesterone the risk of endometrial cancer increases eightfold." Very often the next thing I hear is, "I'll keep the sweats and do without the period."

Rapid estrogen withdrawal by itself is likely to cause hot flushes, which is the reason why many gynecologists prescribe use of the transdermal estrogen patch immediately following surgery for patients who have undergone a hysterectomy with removal of both ovaries. In women who have had a hysterectomy and thus have no uterus to worry about, we can give estrogen alone, but for the rest, progesterone must be added to protect the uterus from cancer.

The progesterone is in a synthetic form, known as a progestin. The common progestin given in hormonal replacement therapy is medroxyprogesterone acetate (MPA), or Provera. There are three types of naturally occurring estrogen: estrone, estradiol, and estriol. Estradiol is the principal and most active form of estrogen. Ethinyl estradiol is one of the most potent synthetic estrogens. (The estrogen preparations listed in Table 5 include brand names. The patient should be aware that similar doses of generic preparations of estrogens have been reported not to relieve menopausal symptoms.)

There are three recommended regimens for hormonal replacement therapy. The standard approach is for the patient to take estrogen for the first 25 days of the calendar month, and for days 13 through 25, progesterone is added; on days 25 through 30, nothing is taken, and that is when the bleeding occurs. A less common

approach is to give estrogen for the entire 30 days, with progesterone added during the first 12 days. This approach is usually
used for women without a uterus, but it can also be used in women
with their uterus intact. In the third regimen, the estrogen and
progesterone are taken at the same time for the entire 30 days.
Endocrinologically speaking, this is probably the best way and I
try to persuade patients to give it a prolonged try, but there may
be spotting and bleeding throughout the month for two or three
years, and, practically speaking, most patients just find it too
antithetical to their lifestyle. They would prefer predictable, cyclic
bleeding with the standard approach rather than the unpredictable,
although lighter, bleeding associated with the combined, continuous
estrogen–progesterone regimen. Each woman is different. One form
of estrogen replacement may be effective for one woman but ineffective for another. Also, one type of estrogen may cause side-effects
that another type may not, which should prompt a change in either
the type of estrogen medication prescribed (for example, Premarin
versus Estratab) or the route of administration (oral versus patch).

TABLE 5.

Postmenopausal Hormonal Replacement Therapy

Type	Dose
Oral Estrogen	
Premarin® (conjugated estrogens), mainly estrone; commonly used in U.S.	0.625–1.25 mg, daily
Estinyl® (ethinyl estradiol) commonly used in Europe	5–10 mcg, daily
Estrace® (micronized estradiol)	1–2 mg, daily
Estratab® (esterified estrogen)[a]	0.625–1.25 mg, daily
Ogen® (estropipate)[b]	0.625–1.25 mg, daily
Transdermal Estrogen	
Estraderm® patch (estradiol)— Ciba	0.05–0.1 mg, twice a week
Climara® patch (estradiol)— Berlex	0.05–0.1 mg, once a week

Type   *Dose*

Estrogen Cream

Estrace® 0.01% (estradiol)
Premarin® 0.0625% (conjugated estrogen)[c]

Combination

Estrogen and progesterone: Prempro® (conjugated estrogen and medroxypprogesterone—MPA)	0.625 mg estrogen with 2.5 mg MPA, daily
Estrogen and androgen: Estrace® (esterified estrogen and methyltestosterone—MT)	1.25 mg estrogen with 2.5 mg MT, daily

[a]Principally estrone of the type excreted in the urine of pregnant mares.
[b]Estrone that is now prepared from the Mexican yam (*Dioscorea*) rather than from the urine of pregnant mares.
[c]A mixture of estrone and equilin prepared wholly or in part from equine urine, or prepared synthetically.

Side-Effects and Contraindications. A patient with unexplained vaginal bleeding, breast cancer, or melanoma should not be taking estrogen replacement therapy. Other contraindications are cirrhosis of the liver, a history of blood clots in the legs or lungs, and, of course, pregnancy. Another concern about estrogen replacement therapy is that a postmenopausal woman taking estrogen is almost three times more likely to develop gall bladder disease and gallstones than a woman not doing so.

Because birth control pills and estrogen replacement therapy both contain estrogen, many people confuse the side-effects associated with the birth control pill with the same potential side-effects of postmenopausal estrogen replacement therapy. However, the usual daily dose of conjugated estrogen, such as Premarin, is three to five times *lower* in potency than the estrogen (usually ethinyl estradiol) in the Pill. Therefore, the frequency and severity of side-effects from estrogen in postmenopausal estrogen replacement therapy is much lower than those that may be experienced with the Pill. Adverse side-effects of postmenopausal estrogen replacement therapy are infrequent; they are listed in Table 4.

For premenopausal women who have had a total hysterectomy

and removal of both ovaries, estrogen replacement therapy not only helps with relief of hot flushes but also reduces the incidence of vaginal dryness and painful intercourse (dyspareunia). But estrogen alone may be woefully inadequate to maintain the libido. For this purpose, androgen (methyltestosterone) is used and has proved to be effective. It can have the side-effects of acne and deepening of the voice, however. Androgens are also being considered for use in post-menopausal women. The FDA has approved Estratest as the androgen-containing hormone replacement therapy in the United States, but published studies suggest that the addition of androgen to a postmenopausal estrogen replacement regimen is no more effective in enhancing sexual drive or reducing depression than the standard estrogen-only therapy. Androgen may place the postmenopausal woman at higher risk for heart disease because of its adverse effect on the "good" cholesterol, HDL, and prolonged use can result in fluid and sodium retention, as well as liver dysfunction. Androgen use with estrogen replacement therapy also has not been shown to have the same bone-sparing effect seen with estrogen use alone.

Posthysterectomy. The woman who has had a hysterectomy without removal of her ovaries may turn up in her gynecologists's office at age 48 or 50 saying, "Gee, what's going on?" The answer is: "You're going through menopause, but you can't see it because you don't have your period anymore."

"What are we going to do about these miserable hot flashes?"

"You can have estrogen replacement therapy."

"No, that causes cancer."

"Of what? You don't have your uterus, so what are you going to have cancer of?"

"Doesn't estrogen cause breast cancer?"

I admit that recent studies have shown that estrogen alone, without progesterone, slightly increases the risk of breast cancer.

"But," I ask the patient, "are you willing to go through years of hot and cold flashes and night sweats when the likelihood of your getting breast cancer is very, very little different from that of the general population?"

The fact is that all of us are at risk for breast cancer until we die; there is no peak incidence as there is for cervical cancer in our 30s and uterine cancer in our 40s and 50s. Thus, I cannot promise this patient that she will not get breast cancer; but if she does, it may have little or nothing to do with the estrogen therapy. I can only tell her that if she is willing to do a breast self-examination each month to detect the first sign of trouble, the benefits of estrogen therapy will tend to outweigh the risks and make her life a good deal pleasanter.

THE AGING PROCESS

Heart Disease and Stroke. After menopause, there is increased activity of some clotting factors, especially Factor VII. The hyperactivity of this clotting factor may contribute to the increased risk of coronary heart disease in the postmenopausal woman.

With the medical community showing more interest in menopause, there will soon be a plethora of medical studies and investigations on all aspects of menopause. One must be very careful in believing everything one reads on the topic. Many investigators may be biased toward emphasizing certain "newsworthy" aspects of a study while downplaying or totally ignoring other findings that can have a great impact on health. A case in point is an article published in the *New England Journal of Medicine* on August 15, 1996, and reported the same day in the *New York Times* which concluded that women who took estrogen and progesterone replacement therapy had a marked decrease in the risk of coronary heart disease compared to those who had not taken hormonal replacement therapy (HRT). This report sent many women flying to their gynecologists for HRT. However, if one looked critically at the study from an epidemilogical point of view, the study also found that there was a statistically significant *increase* in stroke in women taking HRT! Therefore, as an intelligent consumer, a woman has to decide between an increased risk of stroke or a decreased risk of heart attack with HRT use. A family history of either disorder would be useful in helping the patient to arrive at a decision.

Depression. A naturally occurring amino acid known as tryptophan is decreased in its free or unbound form in the blood of postmenopausal women. Tryptophan is involved with the metabolism of serotonin, and any alteration in tryptophan levels can result in depression. Because of low estrogen levels during the menopause, a woman may be even more predisposed to depression.

Skin Changes. Decreased estrogen levels result in less collagen, the main supportive protein of the skin. Skin thickness decreases about 1–2 percent each year after the onset of menopause. The skin of a postmenopausal woman is less elastic, more transparent—blood vessels are more readily visible—and bruises more easily. The vaginal epithelium undergoes the same changes and is more prone to trauma or infection as a result of atrophic vaginitis. Symptoms may be a burning or itching sensation in the vaginal area or increased irritation when wearing close-fitting underwear.

Painful Intercourse. Because I am a woman, it is easy enough for me to close the door of the office or examining room and say to a menopausal patient, "How is your sex life?" Male gynecologists are less likely to ask the question because they are afraid of sounding intrusive or leering, so unless they know the patient well or unless the patient herself brings it up, which many women hesitate to do, it is a topic that gets passed over. This is too bad because the answer I very often hear is: "It's lousy. It's so hurtful and painful." These are the symptoms of atrophic vaginitis. A two- to three-week course of estrogen cream applied to the vulva and in the vagina can correct the vaginal atrophy and relieve painful intercourse.

Intercourse can also be painful for menopausal women because, in addition to the tissues being thinner and drier, vaginal secretions are decreased. Although sexual response is intact after menopause, the time from sexual stimulation to the time it takes to achieve vaginal lubrication may be as long as five minutes, compared to the 15 to 30 seconds it takes in a young woman. The answer to this awkward annoyance is often as simple as lubrication with Astroglide (see chapter 1) and a little patience from her partner. If lubrication does not work, an estrogen cream applied topically to the vagina can be effective in plumping up the tissues. It is absorbed just as effectively as estrogen taken by mouth, which means that if the patient is going to use the cream for more than a few weeks the protective medication, progesterone, must also be taken, which, as noted, may reinstitute the patient's periods.

There is no reason in the world for a woman's sexual life to end, or even diminish, when she is menopausal. Indeed, she can remain sexually active until she dies, and the more active she is, the fewer problems she will have with sexual relations.

Osteoporosis. As with birth control pills, different patients react in different ways to hormones. Unless the dosage is carefully adjusted and unless the doctor is understanding and encouraging, most women will not refill the prescription, or perhaps even have it filled in the first place. This is an acceptable choice for women of color or hefty women with dense bones because they are not particular candidates for osteoporosis, but for slight women or Asian women weighing in the neighborhood of 100 pounds, it is a disservice not to emphasize to them that the medication is being offered not just to offset hot flashes but to stave off the osteoporosis that leads to bone fractures and disability. If the patient understands this, she may consider the side-effects of hormone therapy worth it, as indeed she should. (See Table 6)

TABLE 6.

Risk Factors for Postmenopausal Osteoporosis

Underweight
White or Asian ethnicity
Family history of osteoporosis
Low calcium intake
Sedentary lifestyle
No children
Early menopause or removal of both ovaries
Alcohol abuse
Cigarette smoking

Estrogen is a powerful hormone that affects the ability of bones to absorb calcium, the mineral that keeps bones strong. The hormone is rather like a carrier pigeon that escorts the calcium to where it should go, and when it is not present in sufficient quantity, the calcium does not go where it is supposed to and the bones start to demineralize. Taking calcium by mouth helps because there will always be some estrogen in the body, manufactured by the adrenal gland—menopause does not mean total absence of estrogen, only that it is significantly decreased—but it may not be sufficient for women who are at risk. It should be remembered that a dose of *at least* 0.625 milligrams of oral estrogen (Premarin or its equivalent) is necessary to protect against bone loss.

If a patient seems a possible candidate for osteoporosis in that she says, "I don't like milk and I sit all day because I'm a secretary," but she adds that she does not particularly want hormone replacement therapy, I ask her to go to a radiologist and get a dual energy X-ray absorptiometry study of her spine or hip. If this X-ray shows normal density of the bones, I agree that she need not have hormone therapy—and we will repeat the X-ray once a year to make sure she remains within normal limits and is not courting a hip or vertebral fracture. If the patient does appear to be at some risk but still balks at hormone therapy, there is a new nonhormonal medication called Fosamax (alendronate sodium). Fosamax works by inhibiting the activity of the cells that cause bone loss (osteoclasts), thus slowing down the rate of bone loss that occurs after menopause and, in most patients, increasing the bone density. As with any prescription medicine, there may be side-effects. With Fosamax, they include nausea, heartburn, generalized muscle pain, and headache, although such side-effects are usually mild and uncommon. Recently, severe esophageal ulcers or erosion of the esophagus has been reported in patients using Fosamax. In order to prevent such esophageal irritation, patients are urged to take the medication with at least eight ounces of water and are directed not to lie flat for at least 30 minutes after taking the medication.

The argument is often presented that by prescribing estrogen for menopausal women, the doctor is killing two birds with one stone; that is, the medication is not only protective against osteoporosis but against heart disease, which is the greatest killer of women. The flaw in this reasoning is that the progesterone that must be taken along with the estrogen negates some of the positive effects of the estrogen. A more optimal protective regimen may be Fosamax for osteoporosis and a daily baby aspirin (or a regular aspirin twice a week) for heart disease.

Actually, the real protection against osteoporosis begins when one is a teenager because porousness of the bones is the end stage of a long process. Continuing to drink milk after childhood through the teenage years is like putting calcium in the bank to be drawn on later, but, unfortunately, teenagers favor sodas over milk and not many drink the two glasses of milk a day that would allow them to meet more than half their daily calcium needs. (For other sources, see Table 7.) Women resume milk drinking under orders when they are pregnant, but after the fetus has extracted the calcium from their bones and the baby is born, they forget about milk once again. Then they arrive at their 50s and discover through densitometry studies that their bones have become rarefied and dowager's hump is in the offing. To start drinking milk then is better than nothing but the real cure is prevention from an early age. Therefore, conscientious mothers of teenage girls should encourage their daughters to drink milk during these formative years.

TABLE 7:

Dietary Sources of Calcium

Dairy *Milk and Milk Products*	*Calcium (mg) per serving*
Whole milk (1 cup)	290
Low fat -2% (1 cup)	297
Skim milk (1 cup)	302
Buttermilk (1 cup)	285
Goat's milk (1 cup)	326
Sheep's milk (1 cup)	474
Ice Cream, vanilla 10% fat (1 cup)	176
soft (1 cup)	236
Yogurt (plain, low fat) (1 cup) 12 gms. protein	415
Yogurt (fruit varieties) (1 cup)	
9 gms. protein	314
11 gms. protein	383
Half and half 1 tablespoon	16
Sour cream (1 cup)	268
Cheese	
Cottage (1 cup)	108
Swiss (1 ounce)	272

Dairy

Milk and Milk Products	*Calcium (mg) per serving*
Cheddar (1 ounce)	204
Provolone (1 ounce)	214
American, processed (1 ounce)	163
Parmesan (1 ounce)	390

Seafood

Salmon, pink (3 ounces)	181
Sardines, with bones (3.2 ounces)	351
Clam chowder, New England (11 ounces)	150
Shrimp (3 ounces)	170

Vegetables and Beans

Tofu (8 ounces)	244
Spinach, vine (3 ounces)	109
Broccoli (1 spear)	205
Collard greens (1 cup)	358
Radishes, dried (4 ounces)	365
Soybeans, dry roasted (1 cup)	464

Source: Wallach, Leah. *Food Values: Calcium.* Harper & Row, New York, 1989.

On the other hand, whether or not she was a milk drinker as a teenager, not every woman over 45 is at risk for osteoporosis. I recently had a black woman come to see me who was about 5'10", weighed 210, and was 42 years old. "Dr. Thornton," she said, "I want whatever you give women to prevent osteoporosis. I don't want any bone fractures."

"Yes," I agreed, "there's osteoporosis out there. There's hip fractures out there, and they cause a lot of disability and death. But how does that relate to you as an individual? If you were a very thin lady, white, from England or Scandinavia, who just sat in a rocker all day, I could fracture a bone by just looking at you as hard as I am looking at you now. But you are black, you are active, and you are a big woman. The last thing you are likely to develop is osteoporosis."

"The ads on TV say . . ."

"Don't pay any attention to ads that tell you all women are at risk.

Certain body types and certain races are. The rest of us really don't have to worry about it."

Calcium need during menopause is 1200 milligrams per day. After menopause, it increases to 1500 milligrams per day.

POSTMENOPAUSAL BLEEDING

If a woman has had no period for six months and then bleeds, she should seek medical attention immediately because this can be a sign of cancer. But what if it happens after five months or seven months? That depends on how conservative her doctor is. Conservative doctors will ask their patients to come in to be checked if the bleeding occurs after five months with no period, while more casual physicians may say, "Seven months? That's no problem. I'll see you at the regular time." But all doctors agree that investigation of bleeding occurring after one year without it is mandatory.

Equally mandatory is the investigation of irregular bleeding—not the spacing out of periods but bleeding that is happening days apart. Many women think that irregular bleeding signals menopause, but that is not so. Bleeding that is happening every three or four days can indicate the presence of a polyp or cancer and should be evaluated immediately.

PSYCHOLOGICAL FACTORS

It helps to know that menopause is not going to last forever. Eventually, in anywhere from three to ten years, the body will settle down. There will be a level amount of hormones, and one's personal thermostat will stop kicking up and down. It is important to keep that in mind, to know that there are a lot of years ahead that will be smooth sailing hormonally. It has been my observation that the mindset with which women enter menopause has a lot to do with how they get through it. When I had a general practice, I could pick out the women who were going to have problems. The ones who were very dependent on their husbands, did not have much self-esteem, and were demanding of attention had a great deal of trouble coping with menopause, while self-assured women who had work to do, who were busy and content with their lives, had an easier time dealing with it.

As discussed earlier, depression may have a physiologic basis in the postmenopausal woman. However, just as the hormonal imbalance in pregnancy can trigger postpartum depression in someone who has not come to grips with a psychological concern before she became pregnant, so can menopause exacerbate depressive symptoms, mild or severe, in someone with psychological problems. Many women experience mood swings, some feel like they are about to have a nervous breakdown, and a certain proportion have to be hospitalized because of incapacitating depression. Physicians and gynecologists look at the patient's history, and if the patient has previously been troubled by depression or suicidal ideation, they are likely to refer her to a psychologist or psychiatrist and to a support group to see her through a psychologically difficult time, as well as treating her with mood-stabilizing medications and estrogen if that seems indicated.

I have patients who say, "My mother had a bad menopause. My sister had a bad menopause. I just know I'm going to have a lot of trouble."

My answer is: "Are you exactly like your sister or your mother? Do you look exactly like either of them? Why do you think you're going to have exactly the same menopause?"

"Well, it runs in the family, doesn't it?"

"No, it doesn't run in the family. What runs in families is attitudes." I go on to suggest that she look at the bright side. Menopause allows women to reestablish their lives as people. This is a great time for a woman to say to herself, "I've sacrificed for my husband, my children, my career, but now I have a chance to see what else there is to life. I can focus on interests of my own and make a plan and set goals for me." Whatever the interest is, if the patient gets caught up in it, when next I see her, what I usually hear is that, yes, the hot flashes come and go "but I'm too busy to pay much attention to them."

WEIGHT GAIN

Because the metabolic rate of the body declines over the years and because women tend to grow less active in their 50s, weight gain can occur in menopause. But it need not. Again, the mindset is important. Women can say to themselves, "Well, I'm menopausal. I'm getting old. What does it matter how I look?" and let themselves go. Or they can say, "This is a great time because now I don't have the ups and downs of being on a diet for two weeks and then ovulating and pigging out on chocolate and cookies. I can stick to my diet and eat properly, without the cravings I used to have." Some women may still have cravings, but they are not due to changing hormonal levels, and increased exercise should restore balance and fitness. The positive effects of exercise, such as ballroom dancing or tennis, on cardiovascular fitness are well known, and exercise also serves to retard bone loss.

As discussed earlier, during and after menopause, estrogen is still being manufactured in the body by the adrenal gland and from fat. An obese lady will not have as many hot flashes as her thin counterpart, but she is at increased risk for the effects of estrogen on her uterus, i.e., endometrial cancer, because the fat metabolizes a form of estrogen called estrone. Whether she is also at increased risk for breast cancer is hard to say. If you are postmenopausal, fat may actually decrease your risk of breast cancer, according to findings of the National Nurses' Health Initiative, a study that has been followed for the last 19 years; but the women in that study are well educated and knowledgeable about the effects of diet, so the findings may not be generalizable to the female population as a whole.

PREMATURE MENOPAUSE

About seven to ten percent of women have premature ovarian failure. At 37 or 38, their periods cease, and believing they are pregnant, they go to the doctor. When the pregnancy test is negative, the doctor proposes, "I'll give you some progesterone to see if we can prime the pump and get withdrawal bleeding." If that does not work, the next thing is an endocrinological workup. If this shows that the FSH and LH—follicle stimulating and luteinizing hormones—are sky-high, the diagnosis is premature ovarian failure. The biological clock has misread the time, and the woman is having menopause in her late 30s rather than her early 50s.

Women with premature menopause definitely need hormonal replacement therapy. The doctor has to do whatever arm-twisting is necessary, repeating over and over, "You need to have it. You need to have it." The reasons are twofold: osteoporosis and cardiac problems. There will be an additional twelve years in which the woman will be without estrogen, and bone density cannot help but suffer. For the same reason, the woman will be at heightened risk for cardiac difficulties. I am not a strong proponent of hormone replacement therapy, believing that it is better to come to terms with the inevitable rather than try to postpone it, but this is one instance in which replacement therapy is imperative.

"Oops" Babies

When a woman of menopausal age has been six months without a period, she should go to see her doctor, at which point a pregnancy test should always be done. The woman may be affronted, but there are 50-year-old women who do not know they are pregnant until they go into labor. They will say, "I'm putting on weight, but that's menopause. I haven't had my period for four months." When they feel movement, they credit it to intestinal movement. They even rationalize away breast engorgement.

Gynecologists, even gynecological oncologists (tumor surgeons), can also be fooled. When I was at Bethesda, a 52-year-old woman was on her way to surgery for a large ovarian tumor. A screening test for ovarian cancer had given a highly positive result, and because a big mass was obviously present, it did not occur to anyone to do a pregnancy test; the diagnosis was cut and dried. Just before surgery, someone said, "Let's do a sonogram of this 26-week-size tumor to see exactly how we're going to deal with it." What they had to deal with was the egg on their faces because the scan showed a 26-week fetus.

The moral is, if you are 48 or 49 or older, and your period that has been coming every month does not come for three months, see your doctor. Do not just assume that it is menopause setting in. You need a pregnancy test and a pelvic exam to rule out, or in, an "oops" baby. I heard a woman on the radio last night say that she had two sons, 32 and 6 years old. It happens. Women say, "Oh, I know my body better than the doctor does," and they let the weeks go by; then comes the golden trimester, the midpart of pregnancy, and they mildly regret the weight gain but otherwise they feel fine, until the third trimester comes and their feet begin to swell. Then they go to the doctor and they are already 28 weeks pregnant. So, ladies, you may think you are menopausal, but you are pregnant until proved otherwise.

POINTS TO REMEMBER

- Average age at menopause is 52, with the spacing out of periods usually beginning about age 48.
- If menopausal symptoms are disruptive to a woman's quality of life or if she is at risk for osteoporosis, hormonal replacement therapy is indicated.
- Hormonal replacement therapy reinstitutes a woman's periods.
- Slightly built women with small bones are at greatest risk for osteoporosis.
- Drinking milk in adolescence is the best preventive measure against osteoporosis.
- Painful intercourse during and after menopause is remedied with lubricating or hormonal creams.
- Irregular bleeding during menopause and any spotting or bleeding after menopause require immediate investigation.
- The mindset with which menopause is approached is important for how it is weathered.
- Weight gain after menopause is by no means inevitable. Exercise is important for keeping off weight and for prevention of bone loss.
- Every sexually active menopausal woman with an intact uterus should have a pregnancy test if she misses a period, to rule out an "oops" baby.

VI

P.S.

22

IS YOUR DOCTOR QUALIFIED TO SEE YOU?

❧

BOARD CERTIFICATION • FACS • FINDING A GOOD GYNE-
COLOGIST • OTHER INITIALS • LEVELS OF HOSPITALS •
HOSPITAL COSTS • PHYSICIAN FEES • COST OF DRUGS •
HMOS •

Most patients assume that if a license to practice medicine is hanging
on the wall of a doctor's office, the doctor is qualified to treat them.
But that is not the case. For example, I have a license to practice
medicine in the states of New York and New Jersey, and that means
I have carte blanche to practice any kind of medicine and do any kind
of surgery. Suppose I took a fancy to do ophthalmologic surgery, for
which I am totally untrained. There is nothing to stop me; no law
forbids my doing so. The type of medicine I practice is not the state's
concern. All the state is acknowledging by granting me a license is
that I have had four years of medical school plus a year of training as
an intern. I can be an OB-GYN, as I am, but I can if I wish also do
brain surgery or foot surgery or liposuction, treat your stomach ulcer
or take care of your child. Am I qualified to do these things? Of
course not.

BOARD CERTIFICATION

What a patient needs to look for, after seeing the license to practice
medicine on the wall of a doctor's office, is a second document testi-
fying to Board Certification in the doctor's specialty. Indeed, even
more to the point is to ascertain whether the doctor is Board-
Certified when you call initially to make an appointment. Some

receptionists have been instructed to answer yes even if the doctor is not Board-Certified, which is not honorable but it does happen. If you are not entirely convinced by the receptionist's reply, go to a public library. In the reference section will be a *Directory of Medical Specialists*. The names are organized by state and specialty, so that if, for instance, you live in Massachusetts and wish to check whether Dr. X in Boston is Board-Certified in Obstetrics and Gynecology, you can simply run down the list of OB-GYN specialists in Massachusetts. Alternatively, in this same book there will be a telephone number for the American Board of Obstetrics and Gynecology; you can call the number and say, "I want to know whether Dr. X is Board-Certified," and the answer will come back yes or no. Or you can call the American Board of Medical Specialties at (800) 776-2378 to find out about any doctor in any specialty. An operator will tell you whether the doctor is Board-Certified and if so, in what specialty, and the year he or she obtained Board Certification.

The reason I stress Board Certification is because doctors can call themselves infertility specialists or perinatologists or anything else they please. They are not compelled to undergo further training in a specialty in order to practice it. Only Board Certification confirms that they have had the training. A doctor, when asked, may answer, "I'm Board-eligible," or "I'm Board-active," but anything other than the term *Board-Certified* means that the doctor is not a qualified specialist.

The Board Certification process is a voluntary examination that is comprehensive and exhaustive. Usually given in two parts, it tests the candidate's didactic, or book, knowledge and the clinical application of this knowledge. To take OB-GYN as an example, the written part of the examination is taken in June of the last year of a four-year residency in obstetrics and gynecology. Passing the written examination means that half of the process for becoming Board-Certified has been accomplished. The resident, now called an attending physician, then goes out into practice and sees patients. For the second part of Board Certification, which comes about two years later, the candidate assembles a list of patients he or she has treated, and from that list selects a number to present to the Board.

For example, I, the applicant, list 40 hysterectomies I have done and give the histories. One such history might be: "The patient came in with heavy bleeding, and on examination was found to have a

20-week-size myomatous uterus." If I then say that I gave the patient a prescription for estrogen, I fail the test because that is the wrong treatment. What I do say is: "I did a pregnancy test, an ultrasound examination, and a hysteroscopy or D and C. The patient continued to bleed and a hysterectomy was performed. The pathology report showed . . ." The Board then questions me about details of the management of the case. What the Board is interested in is how I as the applicant apply didactic theory to the clinical management of patients.

The Board is comprised of directors of training centers and esteemed professsors at teaching hospitals and medical centers across the country. The candidate sits before this august battery of professors and directors and is asked questions, not just about the case list presented but about hypothetical cases as well. "What if a patient presents with . . . ? How would you handle a situation in which . . . ?" "Review these slides and tell us whether you agree or disagree with the pathologist's diagnosis." This oral examination, which lasts a couple of hours, is rigorous. Passing it means that you have been found to be qualified as a specialist in your field.

If I were a patient, I would want to be certain that the doctor treating me has the skills that Board Certification attests to. If you ask whether the doctor is Board-Certified and the answer is no, the next question is: "How long has the doctor been in practice?" If the answer is, "Fourteen years," you know the opportunity has come and gone for this person to be Board-Certified. On the other hand, if the answer is that the doctor is just out of a residency program, it does not matter in the least that he or she is not yet Board-Certified. That will come later, and in the meantime you will benefit from the most up-to-date medical knowledge. When a doctor passes the Board Certification process, he or she is then a diplomate of the American Board of the particular specialty.

There are a lot of doctors but you have only one body so you should choose the best caretaker you can find for that body. If you move to another town and must find a new doctor, it may happen that your chemistry and that of the only Board-Certified doctor do not mesh too well and you are tempted to switch to the other doctor in town who is suave, drives a Mercedes Benz, and plays tennis at the country club but is not Board-Certified. Don't change. Stay with the doctor who is Board-Certified. He may not remark on how becoming your dress is, but he will know the right management decisions to make. A nice and compassionate doctor is a pleasure. A highly competent doctor is a necessity.

Board Certification is available in every field, from family practice to OB-GYN to orthopedic surgery to psychiatry to internal medicine, and the document on the wall is quality assurance for the patient, as are such letters after a gynecologist's name as FACOG, which means that he or she is a Fellow of the American College of Obstetricians and Gynecologists, a further step for which the doctor becomes eligible after passing the Boards. Not all Board-Certified doctors choose to accept the invitation to join the college of their specialty, but most do because the college supplies updates on what is going on in the world of that specialty, and when you are out of training, it is an important source of current information.

FACS. General, orthopedic, gynecological, and ophthalmologic surgeons, when Board-Certified, become Fellows of the American College of Surgeons, which is not broken down into subspecialties. Folks like me who have both FACOG and FACS after their names have not only been Board-Certified in obstetrics and gynecology but have passed strict requirements to become Fellows of the American College of Surgeons. Again, in a voluntary procedure, one goes before an august body of surgeons to be tested and interviewed to determine whether one's surgical skills are appropriate to one's specialty. A case list is generated of all patients the candidate has operated on in the previous two years, and he or she is questioned on both this list and on hypothetical cases: "What would you do in this case? What kind of procedure would you use? What technique would you employ?" Some doctors say, "I'm an FACOG, I don't need to do all that stuff," but I want my patients to know that I am not only a specialist in maternal/fetal medicine but that I have passed the scrutiny of surgeons as well.

The acronym *FACR* is what you should see when you go to a radiologist's office for, say, a mammogram. It means that the radiologist has been accredited by the American College of Radiology. If radiologists have certification in mammography, they are proud to display the FACR certificate, and if as a patient you do not see it, it should give you pause.

So should the absence of an FACP certificate in the office of a family practitioner. If the doctor is a Fellow of the American College of Physicians, he or she is Board-Certified in family and general practice and internal medicine. "I see the M.D. and that's enough for me," patients say, but they are 20 or 30 years behind the times. The medical profession is now policing itself, and patients should take advantage of that to make sure they are getting the best care.

Finding a Good Gynecologist. Friends can be a wonderful source of information, but check their recommendation of a gynecologist at the library because they may be basing their judgment of a doctor on manner rather than qualifications. Patient satisfaction surveys ask: Did the doctor smile? Was the room attractive? Did you have to wait long? But these fade in importance when the doctor is going to deliver your baby or operate on you.

On the other hand, nothing says that a smart doctor cannot also be compassionate. If the doctor has a personality that does not lend itself to a satisfying interaction with patients, he or she should be in a laboratory working with rats. Board Certification does not guarantee personality, and if the chemistry between you and the doctor is not good, you should be on the lookout for another Board-Certified doctor with whom the chemistry is better. You want someone who is both knowledgeable and compassionate if at all possible—that is, if your choice is not limited by geography.

You also want someone who is available. You don't want to be told, "He'll get back to you," and never hear from him. Or, "She's too busy to see you any time soon," and you have to wait weeks for an appointment. If doctors are that busy, they should cut back on their practice or get other doctors to join them in it. Knowledgeable, compassionate, available, that is what you as a patient need in a physician—and in a pinch you can do without compassionate. But never settle for compassionate in the absence of the other qualities because if a doctor goofs up on your body, he or she goes on to another patient but you cannot go on to another body.

OTHER INITIALS

While "M.D." after a physician's name stands for "doctor of medicine," "D.O." stands for "doctor of osteopathy." People often, mistakenly, think a doctor of osteopathy is not a real doctor. In fact, he or she is trained in the same fashion and to the same degree as doctors of medicine; there is no distinction between them.

Osteopathy is a system of therapy based on the theory that the body is capable of making its own remedies against disease and other toxic conditions when it is in normal structural relationship and has favorable environmental conditions and adequate nutrition. M.D.'s tend to be snobbish about D.O.'s, but this attitude is a holdover from the old days when schools of osteopathy emphasized treatment of the skeleton and muscles. Now the medical training is indistinguishable, and a D.O. is the same as an M.D. to all intents and purposes. Board Certification and becoming a fellow of the college of their specialty is equally available to both.

"D.C." after a person's name is a different matter. The letters stand for "doctor of chiropractic," and that is not a doctor of medicine. You will sometimes see "Chiropractic Physician" or "Chiropractic Surgeon" on the shingle outside a chiropractic office, but the practitioner is not a physician and not a surgeon. Chiropractors are limited in their training and in their understanding of the ills that flesh is heir to. Chiropractic is based on the theory that disease is caused by interference with nerve function; what chiropractors do know about is manipulation of the spinal cord. Orthopedists work closely with chiropractors, just as obstetricians work closely with midwives, but like midwives, chiropractors are in an ancillary profession.

The acronyms P.A. and P.C. are other initials that may appear after a doctor's name, and I have heard patients say, "Well, my doctor is a P.A." or "My doctor is a P.C." But the initials have nothing to do with medicine. The former stands for "professional association" and the latter for "professional corporation," and both are tax shelters. They mean that the doctors work for their practice as employees. You would suppose that a doctor might be embarrassed to advertise that he is in a tax shelter, but if patients do not know what the initials mean, they sound impressive. Because the tax laws have been changed recently and P.C. is not quite the tax shelter it used to be, the vogue letters now are L.L.P., standing for "limited liability partnership"; again, they have nothing to do with medicine.

Other initials you may see after a medical professional's name are: R.N., "registered nurse"; L.P.N., "licensed practical nurse"; C.N.M., "certified nurse–midwife"; and M.P.H., "Master of Public Health."

LEVELS OF HOSPITALS

There are level one, two, and three hospitals, also called primary, secondary, and tertiary care hospitals, and designated as such by the state. It would seem that a level one hospital should be the best, but actually level one is a community hospital handling uncomplicated cases and routine procedures. Level two is the next step up and indicates that the hospital can do more complicated procedures. For instance, it can handle transfusions, has an intensive care unit for cardiac problems, and has a nursery to take care of sick babies, although not very, very sick babies. Level three, or tertiary care, hospitals are the big medical centers that can do such things as heart and liver transplants; they are staffed by megaspecialists and microspecialists, and they are where you want to be if you have a tough problem.

When you are having a baby, not everything, as this book has tried to make clear, is predictable. The likelihood is that the course of pregnancy, labor, and delivery will be uneventful, in which case the community hospital with its manicured grass, attractive rooms, and hot and cold running nurses will meet your needs beautifully. But if your baby is sick, is the baby going to stay with you at that hospital? If you ask this question and the answer is no, if they say, "We send them to X hospital," then X hospital is perhaps where you should be in the first place. The hard and tough question is: "If the mother is really sick and the baby is delivered at 26 weeks into the pregnancy, can they be taken care of in this hospital?" If not, the next question is, "Where are they taken care of?" If that hospital is really far away, okay, you take your chances, but if it is reasonably convenient, you have a decision to make.

Some doctors have dual privileges—at both level one and level three hospitals. If not, perhaps the doctor has an associate who does. If you like your doctor and want to stick with him or her but he or she does not have privileges at the major medical center, you can ask which doctor he or she turns their patients over to and ask to meet that doctor. If he or she does have dual privileges, you can stipulate that you would prefer to preregister at the level three hospital. That hospital will have a neonatal intensive care unit and perinatalogists on staff. Alternatively, you should make sure that the hospital you will be going to has a mechanism in place whereby immediate transfer—for instance, by helicopter—is available if needed. If trouble is foreseen, if the pregnancy is complicated, what we call an *in utero* transport is preferable—that the mother and baby come as a unit to the level three hospital before the baby is born.

The level three hospital can come as a bit of a shock to a patient transferred from an attractive community hospital because tertiary care hospitals are not particularly concerned with aesthetics. They are concentrating on, "Is the ICU ready? Get the IV in! Get the scope!" As a perinatologist at such a hospital, I can testify that we are not worried about the fluff; we are out to save the patient's life. The patient is here because she has a problem, and we work to solve that problem.

Hospital Costs. You may wonder why a hospital room costs as much per day as the presidential suite at the finest hotel in the land. The answer is that you are paying not only for yourself but for three other uninsured patients who come into the emergency room. You are paying for the crash carts, the bandages, the blood transfusions of gunshot wound victims, AIDS patients, abused children, and riders who have been in motorcycle accidents, as well as people who do not have a doctor of their own and use the emergency room as a clinic. In the past ten years, the emergency aspect of hospitals has gone up 10 to 20 percent, while inpatient elective stays have gone down by at least an equal amount. If the federal government really wanted to do something about health care costs, the place to assign funds would be to emergency rooms and insuring the uninsured. Actually, if it were up to me, I would set up satellite clinics run by the United States Public Health Service, staffed by residents who have had loans to attend medical school, to treat people who are uninsured. Charity care is the responsibility of all citizens; hospital patients should not be the only ones taxed for it.

Physician Fees. I know that many patients feel that doctors' fees are too high, but the truth is that the physician's share of the health care dollar has consistently remained around twenty cents. In contrast, hospital charges, the cost of expensive medical technology, and the administrative overhead of insurance companies have skyrocketed. It may be that physicians' fees are still too high, but Tiffany doctors do not come at K-Mart prices.

To illustrate what the view is like from the other side of the examining table, let me tell you about an obstetrical patient who had a multitude of serious problems during her pregnancy. She remarked casually, "That's what I'm paying you for—to take care of them."

"Excuse me?" I said. "I pay my gardener more than you're paying me. You can't pay me enough for the ultimate responsibility I have for you and your child, for the fact that whenever you need me, I'm there, for the inconvenience you cause me and my family when you call on a Sunday afternoon or at two or three in the morning." I was really upset. "Six thousand dollars is nothing for a full nine months of total, uninterrupted, devoted care from a high-risk perinatologist!"

Ironically, the woman was a lawyer, and lawyers charge for every minute of their time, but she was unsympathetic to the notion that there is no way to put a dollar sign on the time a caring doctor spends with a patient in trouble.

When the patient went into labor at two o'clock in the morning, I was there. "I'm sorry I had to call you at this hour," she said, a bit sheepishly.

"Your waters broke, we're here, let's have at it." I stayed with her throughout the night. By two o'clock the next afternoon she was only at 3 centimeters. She slowly progressed throughout the day. At ten o'clock that night I was still by her side. It was four o'clock the next morning when I delivered her baby by cesarean section because the fetal heartbeat had gone down. At her postpartum visit, she started to leave, then turned back at the door to say, "Now I understand. The hours you spent with me, the hours you spent with my baby, the way you pulled us both through—no amount of money can pay for that. You were right, and I'm so sorry I said what I did."

Now it was my turn to be sorry that I had blown up at her, but I did not regret that I had let her know that doctors have feelings, that it is not all cut and dried and "How much money can I make out of this patient."

Cost of Drugs. Another troubling thing for patients is the cost of brand-name drugs. Again, it is not simply a ripoff by the pharmaceutical companies, as so many patients seem to believe. There is such a thing as bioavailability. A generic drug may be chemically the same as the brand-name drug prescribed but not be available to the body in the same way and not have the same quality assurance. Take ibuprofen versus Motrin. The chemical is ibuprofen, but the maker of Motrin has formulated its ibuprofen to dissolve and get into the system quickly, while the generic ibuprofen may be compressed into a tablet that sits in your stomach for an hour and a half. There has been extensive testing of the brand-name drug to make sure it does the job it is intended to do, which is not to say that the generic drug is bad, only that it may not have the same effectiveness.

For instance, because a gynecological infection is so deep in the pelvis, it is necessary to hit it hard, hit it fast, and hit it with the right antibiotic, one that has been tested and its bioavailability established, so I may write a prescription for Vibramycin. The patient goes to the pharmacy and is told it will cost two dollars a pill. She all but faints, so the pharmacist says, "You can have doxycycline instead, the generic version; it is only one dollar a pill." One dollar a pill is still a lot, but the patient decides she has to have it, takes it faithfully, and comes back to me in a month—still with the infection. Because treatment failures really bother me, I hunt for the reason. "Let's go back to the beginning. What did the pharmacist actually give you?"

"He said the generic is just the same."

It is not just the same. The pill has not been formulated to get to its target and do its job. Better to have bought the brand name in the first place than be stuck with the infection and perhaps develop an additional yeast infection from the inadequate antibiotic treatment.

For medications that have been around for a long time, like penicillin or Lasix, a generic version is fine, but for things like arthritis or pain medications and the antibiotics, it is important to stick with the brand names that have been formulated for specific results. It may seem that the pharmacist is being altruistic when he offers to save you money by filling your prescription with a generic drug, but he is likely to have paid $1.95 a pill for the brand-name pill that sells for $2, giving him a profit of 5 cents, while he has paid 75 cents for the generic, giving him a profit of 25 cents. He is happy to sell you the generic, but you are apt to feel better faster with the brand name.

HMOs

Since doctors have the ultimate responsibility for a patient's life and well-being, it is doctors who should be making the decisions about the patient's care. But these days health maintenance organizations are making the decisions. Granted that when patients had health insurance, doctors often abused it, but at least it was with the patient's best interests at heart. A doctor would say, "I don't know whether she absolutely needs this chest X-ray, but her lungs sound a little dull, so I guess we'd better have it done to be on the safe side." Currently, the chest X-ray may well not be ordered because if it is, the doctor will be economically penalized for it.

This is referred to as shifting the risk. But it is not the medical risk—that is shifted on to you, the patient—it is the financial risk. The insurance company shifts it on to the doctor—the more procedures he or she orders, the less money he or she makes—and the doctor shifts it on to you, although you may not realize it because the doctor may not mention that he is weighing the necessity of a lung X-ray. If you do become aware of it, you can decide to pay for the X-ray yourself, which means that the financial risk has been shifted on to you, and that is where the other two parties are content to have it.

The doctor is not going to be explicit about this, of course. He will say, "Well, I don't think you really need an X-ray. Let's wait another couple of weeks and see if things don't clear up by themselves." And, yes, they might clear up, but if your doctor is part of an HMO, you should always have it in mind that there may be a conflict of interest for him or her between your health and his or her financial return.

If you are an employee in a large company, chances are you will be forced into an HMO because the company does not care about the quality of the health care as much as it cares about the cost of coverage for its employees. An article in the *New York Times* surveyed what company executives have in the way of health insurance, and it turned out that although they pay the same amount in premiums, they are not in HMOs; their insurance covers fee-for-service health care. If HMOs are so great, why aren't they great for the executives as well as the workers?

The stock of the large HMOs is publicly traded, which translates to the fact that the management's first responsibility is not to patients but to the stockholders. If you are a member of an HMO, you are "a covered life," and "covered lives," like "pork bellies," are a commodity. If you wonder why your HMO premiums are not that much different from those of the old indemnity insurance, it is because HMOs are in business to keep their stockholders happy and pay their CEOs salaries in the millions of dollars. No matter what you think of the old health care system and doctors driving around in Mercedes, most of the money found its way back into health care: doctors enlarged their offices, they bought new and better equipment, they added to their staffs. Now the money is going into the pockets of people who are going to buy boats and condominiums with it. That is what irks doctors. The HMO tells us that it is not going to reimburse a patient for a three-day hospital stay we know is necessary and then pockets the money and the CEO vacations in the south of France.

The people running the insurance companies are great in business, great at cost containment through denying claims, but people are not the products of an assembly line. Each body is different, and unless each is handled individually, some are going to die. But the reasoning of businessmen goes like this: "If you ship light bulbs, there's going to be a couple that break on the way. If you treat everybody the same way and a couple of people die, well, that's business." The HMOs have what is called ADR, an acceptable death rate. For instance, the ADR for a cardiac intensive care unit is two percent. Does an acceptable death rate strike you as an oxymoron? It does me as a physician, but to a businessman it is economics—unless the patient is a family member.

The HMOs have found that the quickest way to make a profit is to cut the length of hospital stays. That shifts not only the financial risk of caring for the patient to the family but it also entails social risk in that taking care of the patient is stressful and may impact upon the employment work-days of other family members. Also, it is putting a lot of hospital personnel out of work, a consequence of having an economic-based approach to medical care versus a humanity-based approach. Is it what we want? Can we change it? Perhaps not, but we changed the old to get here. Why can we not change the new back to some sort of middle way where the patient's health rather than the pocketbook of either the CEO or the M.D. is the focus?

What is being discussed now as a possible answer are POs—physician organizations. These are organizations consisting of over 100 physicians, both specialists and generalists, who assume the global risk for patients much as HMOs do now. The PO will go to a corporation and say, "We can take care of your people for the same premiums you are giving the HMO, but now all the money will go into health care rather than having 11 cents of each dollar go into advertising and marketing as it does now, with further percentages going into overhead, salaries, and profits." The physicians themselves will be, in effect, the insurance company; they will be the ones taking the risk.

They will make a profit, yes, but not huge amounts, not the million dollars a day that an HMO makes, and they will reinfuse money into patient care so there will not be denial of needed treatment on the grounds of its being experimental, as too often happens now. The disincentives of, "If you order that X-ray, your salary's going to be cut," or, "If you order that test, you're going to be deselected," will vanish. The good thing about the rise of the HMOs is that they have taught doctors to be more efficient, but disincentives and threats are terrible ways to practice medicine. The important people in the equation, patients and physicians, need to get together to take control of health care away from the business-oriented people and return it to a humane and relevant basis.

To illustrate that physicians are not unaware of their own need to rethink current medical practices, I would like to end by quoting from a speech I was asked to give before the 42nd Annual Clinical Meeting of the American College of Obstetricians and Gynecologists in May 1994.

I have been asked to speak about "the whole patient," patient education, and patient advocacy. The first thing to be said is that the whole patient is greater than the sum of her parts. As specialists, we have been trained to evaluate, critically examine, and treat "parts"—uteruses, cervices, ovaries, contraction patterns—without taking into account the person who is behind the speculum and up in the stirrups. Having taken our diagnostic skills to a high level, we are startled when patients seem to prefer the advice given by talk show hosts and in the pages of magazines. But how can we blame the patient when we refer to her as "the hysterectomy" in the recovery room or "the preeclamptic" in Labor and Delivery?

I am sure many of us as attendings have witnessed a resident walk into the room of a patient in labor and, with back to the patient, review the fetal monitor tracing, see no evidence of contractions on the monitor, and walk out wondering why the woman is screaming her head off. It is up to us as mentors and teachers to tell the resident to go over to the patient and place his or her hand on the patient's abdomen and feel the contraction. For some residents, this is a revolutionary concept: to actually touch the patient and learn that the monitor is wrong. We have become more concerned with what is going on *in utero* than the whole woman who is *ex utero*. We have to teach our residents that they must become more responsive to the emotional, social, and psychological health of their patients, not just to the clinical aspects of their illness.

The College and many others who are interested in the best in women's health care have fought long and hard for the OB-GYN practitioner to be designated as a primary care physician because the OB-GYN may be the only physician a woman visits for her health care. Statistics show that over seven million women a year will have their general medical examination performed by their gynecologist, which makes it incumbent upon us to perform a thorough examination. We need to have our patients disrobe, not just from the waist down, but entirely, so that we do not do just a pelvic examination but examine the thyroid, abdomen, lymph nodes, and breasts. We must also take the opportunity to review breast self-examination and educate the patient about when to be concerned. And because we are dealing with a whole person, the final part of the examination should be to ask the patient: "Is anyone hurting you?" With this nonthreatening question, we can discover whether the patient is one of the more than six million women abused by their spouses each year. Almost ten percent of pregnant women are victims of domestic violence, and we as gynecologists may be the only person the patient feels comfortable enough with and trusts enough to tell. It can be our chance to help end this terrible epidemic.

It takes time to elicit this information, of course, and many gynecologists feel that their practices have become cattle drives. We as physicians have to fight to reclaim more time with our patients, for we all know that in treating a patient, 90 percent is in the history, only 10 percent in the physical examination. All of us took a sacred oath when we graduated from medical school to practice medicine in the best interest of our patients, not in the best interest of lawyers or HMOs or hospital administrators. We are trained to eliminate infection, treat cancer, and stamp out illness. But a far greater threat to our patients is the erosion of the doctor–patient relationship because of interference from those who do not have the ultimate responsibility for patients' health and put cost-containment above quality assurance.

At present, we have third-party payers dictating care of the patient. As an example from my own practice, one of my patients had a cesarean section and her insurance company mandated her release on the second postpartum day. I told the patient that her bowels must not have been reading the same book as the insurance company because their function had not yet returned. She was so upset over the fact that the insurance company would not pay for an extra day that I called the company's 800 number and waited for a representative to answer the phone. When I got one on the wire, I explained that in my opinion as the attending physician, the patient was not stable enough for discharge because her bowel function had not returned. After a moment of silence, the representative said, "Well, have you given her a suppository?" I couldn't believe my ears—an insurance clerk was telling me how to practice medicine!

In this era of "drive-thru" deliveries when new mothers are being discharged even before their milk has had a chance to come in, we must assume the responsibility of becoming patient advocates. We must not acquiesce to unreasonable demands for shortened hospital stays or avoid performing necessary diagnostic procedures because they are denied by the insurance companies. If we do not fight back, we will not only lose credibility with our patients but our integrity as physicians.

In medicine, we are at a crossroads where our patients are being reduced to CPT codes, invoices, and hospital utilization units. We as physicians must make certain that the humanity remains in medicine. At the same time as we work to make our own relationship to patients caring and concerned, we must insist on the right to provide quality care. If we do not fight for our patients' health and well-being, who will?

BIBLIOGRAPHY

American College of Obstetricians and Gynecologists. ACOG Technical Bulletins and Committee Opinions. Washington, D.C.: ACOG, 1991–1996.

Handbook of Gynecology and Obstetrics. Edited by J. S. Brown and W. R. Crombleholme. Norwalk, Conn.: Appleton and Lange, 1993.

Textbook of Gynecology. Edited by L. J. Copeland. Philadelphia: W. B. Saunders Company, 1993.

Williams Obstetrics, 19th ed. Edited by E. C. Cunningham et al. Norwalk, Conn.: Appleton and Lange, 1993.

INDEX